A Nuts-and-Bolts Approach to Teaching Nursing

Fourth Edition

Mary T. Quinn Griffin, PhD, RN, is an associate professor of nursing at the Frances Payne Bolton School of Nursing at Case Western Reserve University. She received her MEd degree from Trinity College Dublin, the University of Dublin, and both her MSN and PhD degrees in nursing from Case Western Reserve University. Dr. Quinn Griffin has more than 20 years' experience in nursing education in Ireland and the United States. She has taught across a wide variety of nursing programs and has extensive experience in educational leadership. Currently she is teaching nursing theory, educational leadership, research, and genetics courses to Doctor of Nursing Practice students. Her research focus is in genetics and ethical issues related to genetic research. She has expertise in developing strategies for integrating genetics in the nursing curriculum. She is a consultant for the NIH Genetics/Genomics Education Directory, a national resource for faculty to access and facilitate integration of genetics into their curricula and education programs. Dr. Quinn Griffin is a mentor in the Nurse Faculty Mentored Leadership Development Program developed by Sigma Theta Tau International to enhance the personal leadership development of new nurse faculty in order to promote faculty retention and cultivate high-performing, supportive work environments in academe. Dr. Quinn Griffin has numerous publications and presentations.

Jeanne M. Novotny, PhD, RN, FAAN, is dean and professor at the Fairfield University School of Nursing. Her career encompasses more than three decades of leadership in nursing education and administration. Dr. Novotny earned her bachelor of science and master of science degrees in nursing at The Ohio State University and earned her PhD at Kent State University. She holds a certificate from the Harvard University Institute for Management and Leadership in Education. Prior to coming to Fairfield in 2001, she held academic appointments at the University of Virginia, Case Western Reserve University, and Kent State University. Dr. Novotny has taught graduate and undergraduate courses focusing on the nursing care of children, nursing theory, nursing education, leadership, research, and international nursing. She has done international work in Mexico, Chile, and Zimbabwe. Dr. Novotny was elected to the Commission on Collegiate Nursing Education Board of Commissioners and serves on the Commission on Collegiate Nursing Education Accreditation Review Committee. She was a member of the AACN Advisory Board for the John A. Hartford sponsored grant, *Preparing Nursing Students to Care for Older Adults: Enhancing Gerontology in Senior-Level Undergraduate Courses,* and participated in the six Geriatric Nursing Education Consortium meetings that were held across the country. Her current research is focused on creating strategic partnerships that support the preparation of baccalaureate and advanced-practice nurses to improve the care of older adults.

A Nuts-and-Bolts Approach to Teaching Nursing

Fourth Edition

Mary T. Quinn Griffin, PhD, RN
Jeanne M. Novotny, PhD, RN, FAAN

SPRINGER PUBLISHING COMPANY

New York

Springer Publishing Company, LLC
11 West 42nd Street
New York, NY 10036
www.springerpub.com

Acquisitions Editor: Allan Graubard
Composition: Apex CoVantage

ISBN: 978-0-8261-4154-5
E-book ISBN: 978-0-8261-4155-2

11 12 13/ 5 4 3 2 1

The author and the publisher of this Work have made every effort to use sources believed to be reliable to provide information that is accurate and compatible with the standards generally accepted at the time of publication. Because medical science is continually advancing, our knowledge base continues to expand. Therefore, as new information becomes available, changes in procedures become necessary. We recommend that the reader always consult current research and specific institutional policies before performing any clinical procedure. The author and publisher shall not be liable for any special, consequential, or exemplary damages resulting, in whole or in part, from the readers' use of, or reliance on, the information contained in this book. The publisher has no responsibility for the persistence or accuracy of URLs for external or third-party Internet Web sites referred to in this publication and does not guarantee that any content on such Web sites is, or will remain, accurate or appropriate.

A Digital Adjunct is available from textbook@springerpub.com

Library of Congress Cataloging-in-Publication Data

Griffin, Mary T. Quinn.
    A nuts and bolts approach to teaching nursing. — 4th ed. / Mary T. Quinn Griffin, Jeanne M. Novotny.
        p. ; cm.
    Includes bibliographical references and index.
    ISBN 978-0-8261-4154-5 (hardcopy : alk. paper) — ISBN 978-0-8261-4155-2 (e-book : alk. paper)
    1. Nursing—Study and teaching.   I. Novotny, Jeanne.   II. Title.
    [DNLM: 1. Education, Nursing.   2. Teaching—methods. WY 18]
    RT90.N68   2011
    610.73076—dc23   2011020514

Special discounts on bulk quantities of our books are available to corporations, professional associations, pharmaceutical companies, health care organizations, and other qualifying groups.

If you are interested in a custom book, including chapters from more than one of our titles, we can provide that service as well.

For details, please contact:
Special Sales Department, Springer Publishing Company, LLC
11 West 42nd Street, 15th Floor, New York, NY 10036-8002
Phone: 877-687-7476 or 212-431-4370; Fax: 212-941-7842
Email: sales@springerpub.com

Printed in the United States of America by Bang Printing

Contents

List of Tables and Online Resources

The icon ℮ indicates forms that are available online from www.springerpub.com

Preface

To start with, make sure that you have noticed that this book is *not* subtitled "Everything You Need to Know to Teach Nursing." It is meant to be the nuts and bolts of how to teach and a survival manual for those who are teaching for the first time, for those who will eventually work on expanding their knowledge through formal coursework, or for those who are new teachers and need a reference book. It is also intended to be a refresher for faculty members who are reentering teaching, either in the classroom or in clinical settings.

This book will be useful to faculty members teaching in any type of nursing program, from practical nursing to master's programs. Faculty members may find some chapters to be valuable at specific times. For example, if you work with practical nursing students, you do need to consider the variables in assigning patients and supervising students' clinical practice. However, it is unlikely that you would use a seminar approach or that you would require complex written assignments.

The information in this book will be of greatest use to faculty members teaching undergraduate students in associate-degree and baccalaureate programs. Your expectation of students will vary with the level of student. For example, you would not expect a second-year associate-degree student to complete the complex assignments that you might expect from a fourth-year baccalaureate student. We have tried to indicate factors to help you discriminate which assignments would be appropriate for which students.

Because of the practical, hands-on nature of this book, we have avoided a theoretical approach. Lists of resources have been provided for those interested in pursuing specific topics in more depth. Our intention has been to follow Victoria Schoolcraft's practical aspects of teaching and drawing on our own and our colleagues' experiences. If you are searching for something scholarly and theoretical, stop here. Although the chapter titles reflect the previous editions of this book, the contents have been thoroughly revised and updated. New content pertinent to teaching strategies for faculty involved in online teaching including the use of technology in education has been added.

We wish to thank Victoria Schoolcraft, the original author of this book, for the way that she taught faculty to work with students. Her legacy will thrive and continue because faculty responsibilities in the transmission of knowledge intertwined with the roles of practice and research will only become more important in the future.

We would like to acknowledge the contributions of the following students in the Doctor of Nursing Practice program, Frances Payne Bolton School of Nursing at Case Western Reserve University, specifically in the Teaching Practicum course:

Kevin Besse
Connie Chronister
Dawn Columbare
Mary De Hann
Andrea Efre
Alycia Jarvis
Anne Jorgenson
Christina Kalista
Jamie Kitchen
Patricia Sharpnack

It is our hope that you will find the book helpful and encouraging. We also hope that you will love teaching nursing students as much as we do!

Mary T. Quinn Griffin
Jeanne M. Novotny

A Nuts-and-Bolts Approach to Teaching Nursing

Fourth Edition

1

Making Clinical Assignments

S tudent nurses are usually excited about spending time in the clinical setting. Nursing faculty need to capitalize on this excitement and provide the students with the best learning opportunities available during their clinical experience. Students need the clinical setting to apply the knowledge that is gained from classes, readings, group discussions, skills labs, and other learning experiences. If you ask students or graduates what they would change about the nursing curriculum, the majority would proclaim, "More clinical!" This element of the curriculum is essential to the development of critical-thinking skills, student self-confidence, and transformation into a professional nurse.

Once faculty members determine how much time will be spent in the clinical setting, the next step is to determine where the students will go for their clinical experience. Selection of the clinical site is an important task and should be done well in advance of the planned clinical experiences. When selecting the clinical setting, consideration must be given to the learning opportunities available for the students, the availability of experienced registered nurses to work with the students, the location of the clinical setting, transport for the students, and availability of space for meetings and conferences with the students. Many clinical facilities are inundated with requests for clinical placements, and it is increasingly difficult to have all of the clinical experiences close to the academic institution. Many students from the same class may be in clinical groups spread over a wide geographical area, and in some cases, clinicals will be in the evenings. Having students in many different institutions and achieving the same learning objectives pose challenges because the faculty member will need to be familiar with differences among the sites and to address these differences in class. The course faculty is often the coordinator for the clinical teaching for that course and will work with the entire clinical faculty assigned to the course to make sure there is consistency of learning from students across the clinical sites.

Once the clinical settings are selected, the next step is to plan how to make the most use of this valuable clinical time. The key to this process is selecting increasingly challenging patients for students so that, over time, each student gets as much clinical experience and as broad a learning opportunity as possible. To maximize the likelihood of this outcome, each patient selected must provide the student with the opportunity to apply the theoretical information gained from the classroom and other assignments. Every hour in the clinical setting must contribute to the student's ability to learn and master the expected content. This is made possible by the careful selection of patients whose care delivery reinforces weekly learning objectives.

GOALS

The principal goal for the clinical experience is to provide the opportunity for the application of theory and mastery of skills. The most effective clinical settings provide students with an opportunity to practice their psychomotor skills, refine their critical-thinking abilities, and develop their psychosocial skills with actual patients and their families. This process increases students' feelings of confidence and self-esteem and promotes achievement of expected competencies. Self-confidence as a nurse cannot be learned in the classroom. Therefore, gaining self-confidence is one of the most important aspects of the clinical experience.

TOOLS

Course Objectives

The course objectives are the main factors to use when determining which patients to assign to students. If the course objectives relate to caring for patients with simple disruptions in their physical health status, assign patients who match that description as closely as possible. Efforts should be made to assign beginning students in a manner that does not overwhelm them. Because it is difficult in this era to find patients who have simple disruptions in health status, close supervision and support may be required until the student's comfort reaches an acceptable level. In an early clinical course, the faculty member may have no choice but to assign patients with complex problems. The focus of the student actions, however, will be directed toward management of basic needs.

The course faculty should meet with the entire clinical faculty at the beginning of the course and then regularly throughout the course. At the first meeting the course objectives will be presented and plans devised to ensure that there is seamless learning for the students between classroom and clinical teaching. Throughout the course, the faculty will devise additional ways to create learning opportunities that start in the classroom and are completed in the clinical area. Students need to see regular collaboration between the didactic and clinical faculty so they recognize both classroom and clinical learning as interdependent essentials for excellent clinical practice.

Clinical Objectives

In addition to course objectives, faculty should develop detailed clinical objectives that specify the expectations for performance and identify the process of evaluation. These objectives flow from the overall course objectives and link application expectations to knowledge-development components. For example, to identify at least three nursing interventions for a patient at risk for skin breakdown related to immobility, the clinical objectives should state exactly how students would be evaluated when performing psychosocial and psychomotor skills. An acceptable level of competence or skill performance also should be identified. When several clinical faculty members are assigned to the same clinical course, the faculty member teaching the didactic content may be assigned to coordinate the clinical experiences. In this type of situation, all faculty involved in the clinical experience will meet to develop and agree on the clinical objectives, the performance expectations, and the evaluation. Throughout the course, they will meet regularly to discuss student progress. It is vital to have consistency across clinical settings for each group of students.

Student Learning Needs

Course and clinical objectives relate to the learning planned for all the students. In order for each student's needs to be met, however, some modification of additional learning experiences may be required. Differences may exist in the speed at which students learn and in the learning techniques they find most useful. The ability to perform at a certain level may be attained much more quickly by some students. Rather than holding these students back, assign patients that permit them to accomplish new or expanded objectives. Make sure that the registered nurse working with the student knows the student's learning objectives and any particular area that needs improvement.

Give each student as much variety as possible in the types of patients assigned. This includes providing for different medical and nursing diagnoses as well as a variety of demographic parameters. Keep track of this information on a card or notebook with anecdotal notes.

For example, such a record would reflect the efforts made to assign patients with a focus on mobility in the first week. In the second week, a notation would be made about the shift of the focus to problems related to gastrointestinal disturbances. The third week might focus on surgical patients, while the fourth would reflect an assignment related to elderly patients. This record helps make certain that the same kind of patient is not repeatedly assigned to a given student. Keeping a note of the age range and gender of the patients that have been assigned to a student can assist you with future assignments as you try to provide students opportunities with different demographics. It can also help you keep track of the opportunities students have to give medications, do discharge planning, and anything else that meets the student-learning needs for achieving clinical objectives. Also, make notes if there are particular clinical skills that need improvement.

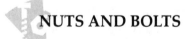

NUTS AND BOLTS

Choosing Patients

Availability

Regardless of what kinds of patients are desired for assignment to students, faculty can only work with the patients who are actually present. Some patients in the census will not be suitable for a variety of reasons. Faculty from other nursing programs or other levels within the same school also may be competing for the same patients to assign. From those patients who are available, the faculty member has to decide the most important things for the student to accomplish and which patient can provide the best experience to achieve that. Faculty may have to give students a patient much like one assigned to them in the past but with direction to focus on something new or more involved than before.

Nurse managers are indispensable in determining which patients to assign to students. They often have information that might encourage or discourage faculty decision making about assignments. Faculty also will have to determine how best to work with the unit manager, while focusing on meeting the individual student's learning needs. Clinical faculty members that are new to the clinical site may wish to spend some time—a few days to a couple of weeks—getting to know the unit routine, the patient acuity, and the policies, procedures, and the staff. This is time well spent, as it will help the faculty member identify learning opportunities more quickly and help foster good relationships with the nursing staff. In addition, faculty should meet with staff a couple of days prior to the beginning of the rotation to let them know about their plans, expectations, the students and their prior experiences, and to hear the staff's expectations for interacting with students and faculty. Faculty members negotiate with the nurse manager about how patient selection will be made. Everything should be done to foster collegial relationships with nursing staff and other health care professionals in the setting. Some nurses on the units will love working with students and will bend over backwards to ensure the learning experience is an excellent one. On the other hand, some nurses do not enjoy working with students, and they may convey this perspective directly or indirectly. It is best to know the nurses that do not want to work with students and assign students to nurses that are willing to work with them. If you are a newcomer, try to rely more on those who like working with students. As you become more comfortable, work on building better relationships with the others and helping them to understand the short- and long-term benefits of interacting regularly with students.

Provide the nurse manager with copies of the objectives that pertain to the clinical experience. The faculty member may like to post a list of things the students are prepared to do and identify those they can do either independently or with assistance. This will remind staff of the types of experiences students are seeking and what aspects of care the students will be expected to perform during the clinical rotation. Often the staff prefers the faculty member to communicate directly with them.

Negotiate with the nurses concerning when to ask for staff input. Some nurses prefer to provide a list that has narrowed down the patient assignment options. This helps to eliminate a patient that may offer suitable learning opportunities but for other reasons is not available for student experiences. Other nurses prefer that faculty make some selections and then provide feedback as needed. With either method of selection, the faculty member should review the patient list with the staff the day before the clinical experience because there may be changes in the patient's condition and therefore the patient may not be suitable for students to provide nursing care. Also, the faculty member should review any recent admissions, because there may be new learning opportunities that have become available. In other words, plenty of time should be allowed for consulting with staff when making assignments. In addition, faculty members must be flexible and accommodate unpredictable or uncontrollable demands on staff time, and staff should review the total assignment to make sure that it is realistic for one faculty member to supervise the range of experiences provided. Often, the most complex patients are assigned because they are the most challenging and provide unique learning opportunities. After faculty and the staff have worked together for a while, adjustments may be made to the original arrangements. Over time, a more give-and-take approach may be possible.

Avoiding Overloading

In a setting that has many student groups, patients may become overwhelmed by the number of students assigned to care for them. Even good students may be taxing to patients. Because students are slower and less certain, they often inadvertently delay or prolong things. This should be considered when making assignments, and periods of non-student assignment may be necessary to allow patients a short-term break. Again, good communication with staff can help avoid these issues. To avoid overloading the patients in the unit, faculty can plan to assign some students to observation experiences. Observation is an important skill for nurses, but students are often overly concerned with doing and do not take the time to observe. Students could be assigned to observe the activity on the unit, or to observe the number of individuals that interact with certain patients in a set time frame. They may also be assigned to observe the leadership role of the nursing manger or the role of the staff nurse. Another observation experience may be to observe experienced nurses performing certain nursing skills.

Multiple Assignments

Although most often one student is assigned to care for one patient, having two or more students working together to care for one patient works well also. Students may be nervous approaching patients during their first clinical rotation and feel safety in numbers when they are in pairs. Assigning student pairs to simply start communicating with the patient helps to build the students' confidence. Although it is appropriate and often a useful experience for more than one student to care for a patient, this may be stressful for the patient. One way to deal with this is to ask the students to review the learning objectives for the day and the plan of care. Get them to plan their nursing care effectively so that each student has an opportunity to provide care. With two students working together, assign both of them to do the physical care, then one to prepare and pass medications and the other to complete procedures such as a dressing change. This process helps students learn collaborative behaviors, and they often find the experience supportive and rewarding. Pairing students also allows the faculty member to team students with different skill levels together. The students can learn from each other, practice collaboration, and begin to develop team-leading skills. It also facilitates the sharing of student learning experience in the clinical postconference.

Assignments

Privacy and confidentiality of patient information are paramount when planning ways to inform students of their assignments for the clinical day. The student only needs to know to what unit the patient is assigned and then make a visit to review the chart prior to the clinical experience.

In some instances, students are unable to or are not expected to complete extensive patient-care planning prior to the clinical day(s). This is particularly true if the student must travel a considerable distance to reach the clinical area. Nonetheless, the faculty member may still want the student to be familiar with the patient. In that case, these expectations should be made clear at the beginning of the course, and all students should be held to the same standards regarding preparation for a patient assignment. Also, faculty may require all the students to have obtained general information such as the most common drugs in use on the unit. Providing the students with details of the learning objectives in advance of each clinical day will help students be prepared.

Student Involvement

As students progress in a course or through the curriculum, the faculty member may want the student to become more involved in selecting patients. One way to accomplish this is to ask students if there are particular types of patients with which they want to work, and then make your assignments accordingly. In doing so, faculty should be certain the students select patients that meet the course objectives, clinical objectives, and individual learning needs. The faculty member could make a list of patients that is greater in number than students and allow students to select from that list. Before trying this option, be sure the nurse manager on the unit understands and agrees with this approach. Another option that may work well with senior students is to have them review the patient lists and select patients they would like to work with as well as one who meets the learning objectives. Ask students to discuss their patient choices with the nurse caring for the patient and also to provide rationale for choosing this patient to you. Assign the patient to the student only after the student consults with the registered nurse and you, and there is agreement about the assignment.

Patient Involvement

To paraphrase Shakespeare, "To ask or not to ask the patient, that is the question." The primary reason to ask a patient about assigning a student is that there might be some reason to think the patient might be reluctant to accept a student. For example, a patient asked that a certain student no longer be assigned to take care of her. When asked why, the patient responded that this had more to do with that particular student than with something generally pertaining to nursing students. The patient was willing to try a different student.

Some faculty members who seem to have no reservations about assigning female students to male patients have qualms about assigning a male student to a female patient. Although some assumptions in this area may be based on bias, it is true that some female patients have concerns about male students being involved with their nursing care.

One way to deal with the assignment of male students is to discuss with the student the possibility of being rejected because of gender. Help the student see the importance of being direct and of conveying confidence when making the initial introduction to the assigned patient.

A female student or nurse may sometimes find it appropriate to request assistance from a male colleague in giving care to a male patient. In any case, discuss this with the patient. All male and female nurses need to understand and be able to provide complete care for both male and female patients.

Other Settings

Psychiatric Units

A typical approach in most programs is to assign one psychiatric patient to each student for the development of an ongoing relationship. Make sure that staff members are clear about what students need to accomplish and clarify those expectations and any restrictions that might affect the goals of the experience.

Community Health

The pattern for assignments in community health is determined by the appropriate focus for a beginning practitioner in this area. One belief is that the focus should be that of traditional public health, which focuses on the promotion of wellness for populations. Another view of nursing in the community looks at care of individuals and families who require care at different levels of prevention and who are outside acute-care institutions. This would include the care of people who have primary prevention needs, such as pregnant women and their families and children, in promoting normal growth and development. It also includes caring for people in their homes who previously would have been cared for in acute-care settings. In the latter example, the care is comparable to medical-surgical nursing in the home rather than in the hospital.

Nonpatient Assignments

In some situations, it is warranted to assign students to do something other than total patient care for one or two patients. In making this decision, faculty should consider whether such an option meets objectives for clinical experience. No matter how much a student would like to tag along with the phlebotomist all day, it would not be a good use of clinical time. On the other hand, such an activity may give the student a perspective of a different pattern for delivering care. Whether or not the activity meets the course objectives should be a determining factor.

When deciding, faculty should look at the quality of the experience in light of the amount of time spent. In order to maximize the use of such an experience, consider giving the student a particular focus for observation. After completing the experience, the student should share with other students what was learned from the focused experience. The student could also be asked to discuss the interpersonal components of the interactions as well as the motor skills involved.

If there are specific deficits in the student's patient-care experiences, rectify the problem by assigning the student to complete certain tasks for a patient rather than providing total care. For example, if students need opportunities to give injections, this could be the focus for the day.

Assignments for short or observational experiences can help to maximize the student's use of clinical time when patients are discharged early or other unforeseen interruptions interfere with the regular pattern of assignments. When this occurs, faculty should expect the student to think through how these experiences relate to the overall clinical component. This might include sharing the experience during a clinical conference, or at least discussing it with faculty.

Evaluating the Process

Midway through and at the end of the course, faculty should evaluate the processes used to assign patients to students, the usefulness of the assignments for meeting course objectives, and the students' assessment of the assignment process and its learning effectiveness. Discussions with students and the unit staff and leadership will help clarify where areas for improvement can be made and which experiences were the most beneficial for the student.

Encouraging students to keep a reflections log that summarizes the day's learning experiences and the way in which the patient assignment facilitated learning may be useful for an ongoing review of assignment adequacy. A review of each day's assignment sheet and faculty anecdotal notes also will provide useful information about how well or poorly the assignment process worked. Using these combined data can be helpful when negotiating possible changes in the assignment process with unit staff and leadership. In all cases, feedback should be provided about the ways in which the students learned best and how the learning environment might be enhanced in the future.

FINAL WORDS

Clinical assignments are one of the unique features of nursing education. The clinical setting allows students to practice skills and to gain the confidence they need for practicing as professional nurses. When patient assignment is done well, students, patients, and staff benefit through the students' increased awareness of the diversity of patients seen and the similarities inherent in a wide range of patient situations.

FURTHER READING

Montgomery, M. (2010). Student self-selection of clinical assignments. *Nurse Educator, 34*(2), 47–48. doi: 10.1097/NNE.0b013e3181990d75
Scanlan, J. M. (2001). Learning clinical teaching: Is it magic? *Nursing and Health Care Perspectives, 22,* 240–246.

2

Supervising a Clinical Group

Supervising nursing students in the clinical setting is among the most rewarding and challenging teaching activities. It is rewarding to observe the students learning and becoming confident professionals before your eyes, but also challenging because you are responsible for the care and skills these students provide during the clinical period. When thinking about supervising students in the clinical area, start by reflecting on personal experiences and feelings. Most people teach as they were taught. If you had a stern clinical instructor who made you feel uncomfortable and on the spot, you may believe that this method is the right way to approach teaching. After all, you turned out pretty well, didn't you?

Although a little anxiety may enhance a student's perceptions and ability to learn, too much is immobilizing and counterproductive. One of the more difficult skills to develop is the ability to achieve the right balance between being the caring faculty member and the concerned nurse. The caring faculty member helps students learn in a supported environment. The concerned nurse monitors the impact of student care on patients and makes certain the patients are not inconvenienced or hurt by novices. Keep in mind that even the clumsiest, least dedicated students do not intend to hurt anyone, and sometimes even the most enthusiastic, dedicated students make mistakes.

The clinical area is the crucible where students combine knowledge with application. It is the sine qua non of nursing education. As a nursing educator, it is your responsibility to help students get as much as they can out of what is a relatively limited experience.

GOALS

Effective supervision of students in the clinical area should foster meaningful learning experiences and ensure safe care for patients or clients. Overall, the goal is to provide the students with excellent learning opportunities and to meet their learning needs while ensuring that all nursing care provided by the students is safe and of high quality.

TOOLS

Course Objectives

The course objectives provide the groundwork for what the students will get out of the clinical experience. If the course is a beginning course in the curriculum, do not expect students to be responsible for complex aspects of patient care. However, even if the course objectives are the most basic, patients may still have complex problems. When supervising students, the clinical faculty is responsible for determining what the students can and cannot do safely. If there are aspects of patient care they will not perform, negotiate with the nurse manager who will be responsible for this.

Course objectives pertaining to clinical are often general, but they should give some indication about the type of patient and the complexity of care with which the student will be concerned. For example, in a basic nursing course, an objective might be, "Identify and implement comfort measures for patients with the following conditions." In a more advanced course, the following objective might be included: "Plan and implement care for patients with multiple system failures."

Clinical Objectives

General course objectives may be detailed into clinical objectives for students to accomplish by the end of the semester. Some faculty members even specify objectives for each week. Most faculty members report that general clinical objectives rather than weekly set objectives are easier to deal with and can be more easily adapted to the patient population. However, when working with beginning students, focus on the steps in the nursing process. Weekly objectives can be written to specify when the students must focus on each step in learning to use the process.

Following is an example of more specific clinical objectives that build upon the course objective: *Identify and implement comfort measures for patients with the following simple medical or surgical problems:*

- Limited mobility
- Dermatological disorder
- Outpatient surgical procedure

Following are examples of clinical objectives related to the course objective: *Plan and implement care for patients with multiple system failures:*

- Give comprehensive care for a patient with failures of at least two systems.
- Care for a patient who is being monitored by at least one type of device.
- Identify the principal effects of the major drugs used with patients in cardiovascular distress.

Guidelines for Clinical Activities

Rather than objectives, give students guidelines for what they are to accomplish, such as when they must complete nursing care plans, when drug cards are to be used, and when they are scheduled to observe a surgical procedure. Written assignments in conjunction with clinical assignments should be handled in the same way as other assignments in terms of their description, submission requirements, and criteria for evaluation.

Nursing Care Plans

Nursing care plans are a standard feature of the clinical experience. However, there is much diversity in care plan formats. It is beyond the scope of this book to deal with the nuances of the nursing process and care plans, but here is a list of some factors to consider in selecting your approach to using care plans:

- Be consistent with the format used by other faculty in your program.
- Be consistent with the theoretical and conceptual values of your curriculum.
- Be consistent with the texts and other readings the students have, or make it clear where and when care plans should vary from those resources.
- Be explicit about what is expected within each step of the plan.
- Match your expectations with the level of the student.
- Be realistic about the amount of information students can read, comprehend, and reorganize into a care plan format in the amount of time allowed. Give minimum and maximum limits on length, depth, and breadth.
- Give clear criteria for the evaluation of care plans and how they contribute to the clinical grade.
- Give ample feedback to help students learn from working out the plans.

Some faculty members expect students to start their care plans before starting the clinical day. These care plans would include the initial parts of the nursing process and provide students with a foundation for the day's activities. Whenever possible, give the student sufficient information prior to the beginning of the clinical day. (This, however, is often not possible because the patient population changes rapidly.)

In some situations, students are not able to go to the clinical area for a planning period prior to the start of clinical. In this case, give them some information about the assigned patients so they have a general idea of what they will need to do for their patients. They might not start their care plans until after they begin to work with the patients.

Be clear with students about the purpose of the nursing care plan. For example, it should be clear if the care plan is a plan for care as well as a report of care given. It is important for students to have this former perception in order to make it clear that the care plan is a valid facet of nursing care. The latter use makes it merely an assignment, which students see as divorced from the real practice of nursing.

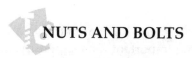

NUTS AND BOLTS

Orienting Students

Orienting Yourself

The school of nursing may assist faculty in getting oriented to the assigned clinical area. If not, arrange this orientation as soon as possible. Find a colleague who has had students in the same agency, especially on the same units where you are assigned. Colleagues can let you in on the way things really work. Some clinical facilities require faculty to attend a formal orientation program prior to taking students into the clinical area. During this orientation program, the faculty may have to demonstrate, or provide evidence of, competency in clinical skills related to the course they are teaching. This program may have additional reading available online, such as policies, procedures, patient safety manuals, and so forth.

Arrange to meet with the staff manager. It is appropriate to start with the nurse manager, but talk with the other nurses as well. Find out what they expect and want from faculty and students. Are there some things they have been particularly concerned about in the past, when they had students? Share the course objectives with them and make sure they know how much the students do and do not know. If they will have to give some aspect of patient care, even if a student is assigned, make sure they understand and agree with what is needed. Discussion with the staff is important because student groups from different programs will be attending this nursing unit for clinical, each with their own needs and expectations. It is easy for the busy staff nurse to forget the expectations you have for your student group in the clinical setting. Be clear in your expectations of your role and the role of the staff nurse taking care of the patient. One issue that comes up a lot from the clinical faculty is that often the staff nurses expect the faculty to provide all the nursing care for the patients assigned to the students. One clinical faculty has approximately 8–10 students; if each student has 1–2 patients, this means the faculty is expected to provide care for as many as 20 patients. This is unsafe and impractical. Ask the nurse manager and staff nurses to tell you how the staff nurses usually work with students and faculty in order to have safe, good quality care. A little reminder: The nursing staff at the clinical agency is responsible for the nursing care of the patients. Spend time getting to know the nursing staff; good communication and a collaborative working relationship are important for a supportive learning environment for the students. This is time well spent.

Preclinical Meeting

Meet with the students prior to going to the clinical area. During this meeting, cover the general things students can expect from the upcoming clinical rotation. For example, let them know what kind of unit they will be working on, the kinds of patients, the staff complement, and what their responsibilities will be. Make sure they all know how to get where they are going, where to park if they are driving, and where to meet when they get there. Tell them what the expectations are for their attire. Encourage them not to bring personal belongings. Many clinical facilities will have a formal orientation for students.

Although your school must provide written policies in a student handbook, it is a good idea to reiterate the pertinent policies every time you start a new clinical rotation. If there is a difference in agency policies and school policies, clarify what the expectations will be for the students. For example, your school may make it optional for students to wear scrubs, but a particular agency may require students to wear uniforms. Make sure the students know if uniforms are required.

Clinical Orientation

Once at the agency, emphasize the information students need to know the most. More complex tours may come later, but to start with, be sure they can get from the door to their unit. Show them around the unit, emphasizing the places they need to know the most about. For example, show them the linen room, the utility rooms, restrooms, places where they can leave their personal belongings, and where they may have access to patient charts. Younger, less experienced students are sometimes so anxious about just being in the hospital for the first time that they may have trouble remembering much of what happens. Make sure they know how they can find you during clinical time. Introduce them to the staff they will work with. Review the role of the staff nurse in their clinical teaching. Make sure they know who to ask if they need help at any time. If possible, arrange for some time for them to meet with the nurse manager or assistant so they can learn about general aspects of the unit.

If the clinical rotation is in a clinic or a community setting, some of the same concerns apply. However, students making home visits require a more extensive orientation. Students are usually nervous about visiting clients in their homes. Give them oral and written information to help them feel more secure. Some of the things to specify follow:

- Proper attire and identification
- Arranging for a time to visit
- Locating addresses
- What to do if no one is at home
- Not to enter a situation that appears unsafe
- To take a companion along when necessary
- Not to transport clients anywhere in their own car
- How clients may contact the student

Prepare a second list that would be more detailed and specific to the agency and the location. The things in the preceding list relate to providing for the students' comfort and safety.

Sometimes, it is possible for faculty to accompany each student on the first home visit. If there are other activities for the rest of the students to participate in prior to their first visits, that is probably the optimal way to start. However, in some situations, faculty may not have the luxury of staggering their starting visits. Another good way to start is for the students to accompany one of the staff nurses on a visit to the assigned client or family. Because home visits are frequently unsupervised by a faculty member, give the students definite parameters for the content and process of the visits. A typical list of guidelines might include the following information:

- Limit the times of each visit to no more than 1 hour.
- Set at least one goal for each visit, but avoid trying to accomplish too much on a visit.
- Let the clients know what the goals are for the visit.
- Encourage the client to ask questions and to help set goals for future visits.
- Clarify for the client when and how goals have been met.
- Include other family members in the interaction when possible and appropriate.

- Use written and pictorial material as well as three-dimensional models to help explain information to clients.
- When collecting data, tell the client what will be done with the information and who will have access to it.
- At the end of the visit, sum up what has been discussed and what the goal of the next visit will be.

Making Assignments

This aspect is covered in detail in Chapter 1. Make certain students know when and where to find out their assignments. Some faculty expect the students to go to the clinical setting the day before they will give care in order to gather detailed information about the client.

Validating Students' Preparation

It is sometimes difficult to check on each student's preparation before you let him or her get started for the day. Students should share the high points of their patients' care in a clinical preconference before they start. As the day goes by, look for opportunities to talk with each student in more depth. Some faculty members expect the students to hand over the beginning of their care plans before they get started.

Occasionally a student is unprepared. If it is the first time this has happened, take the student out of the clinical situation, give him or her time to get prepared, and give the patient back to the staff until the student is ready. Speak with the student about the risks to patient safety when the nurse is unprepared. Ask the student to meet with you once the preparation is completed; if the work is satisfactory, the student can start caring for the patient. Students who habitually come unprepared should be sent off the unit and the day should be counted as an unexcused absence. Check the school policy covering this situation. Document the details of the situation and evidence of repeated occurrences.

Another part of validating preparation is assessing whether the student is physically and mentally ready to care for patients. Some students will stay up so late working on their care plans, or for other reasons, that they are not fit to implement them. Decide if it would be better to send the student home with some words to the wise for better planning in the future. The basis of the student's situation will determine whether or not to count this as an excused or unexcused absence. Make sure you keep accurate documentation of the situation.

Other students may have their functioning altered in other ways, as by drugs or alcohol. It is unfortunate to have to mention this, but it happens. The school of nursing and the clinical facility will have policies for these situations. Make sure you are up to date with the policies. When you have such a situation, you need to act fast and follow the guidelines step by step. These students should always be taken out of the clinical setting, and you need to refer to the policy regarding their return to clinical. Be certain that the specific behavior is documented along with your role in the situation. Report the incident to the nursing program director.

Clarifying Student Roles

It is often difficult to get across to beginning students what they can and cannot do. Some beginning students have done more as nurse techs than they are initially allowed to do as nursing students. They need some help in understanding the role transition. Other students may focus so much on the limits that they cannot see how much latitude they do have. Emphasize to them that they should be conservative, and if they are in doubt, to ask questions. When they are about to make assumptions, the newer they are, the more they need to check their assumptions.

Being a Participant Observer

Acute-Care Settings

In medical-surgical settings, faculty are likely to be involved in helping students in giving care, especially if they are new students. While doing this, be aware that faculty members are serving as a role model. In addition, observe the students' behavior in order to evaluate progress or to identify learning needs.

Develop a style that will enable observation without disturbing the student. Smile and greet both the student and patient when you enter the room. Exchanging a little friendly banter helps to dispel the anxiety the student may feel about being observed.

Participate in the patient's care in a way that feels natural to the patient. For example, if a student seems to be having trouble figuring out how to remove the patient's gown when the patient is connected to an IV, say something like, "That is a tough one. Let me show you how I do it." This conveys to the student that this is just one of those things that takes time to learn, and it keeps the patient from having to worry about what the student is doing.

If the student is about to do something unsafe, such as contaminate a sterile field or administer an injection in the wrong site, try to be as unobtrusive as possible about drawing the student's attention to it. Stop the student verbally if necessary, and try to carry it off so the student does not look or feel incompetent. For example, with a student who is catheterizing a patient and about to contaminate the tip of the catheter, calmly say, "Try holding the catheter closer to the tip. Those things wiggle a lot if you hold them too far down the tubing." This is much less distracting than questions and answers about sterile fields or the physical characteristics of urinary catheters.

When students make errors, talk to them privately as soon as possible about what happened. Encourage the student to analyze what went wrong and to figure out the reasons for it. Discuss ways to prevent errors occurring again. Let the student know that he or she should feel comfortable asking questions when in doubt.

Even with patience and guidance, some students cannot see that they did anything wrong or they cannot think of a correct alternative. Tell these students directly what was wrong and what they should have done. Students like this need close supervision.

Ambulatory-Care Settings

It is sometimes harder to observe students in clinics than in hospital units because it is harder to keep track of where they are. It helps to have a central location where students can leave a note on a clipboard as to which examination room they are in or where they have gone if they have left the clinic.

When and how students are supervised in clinic settings depends upon the purpose of the students' being there. If the experience is strictly observational, the students need guidelines for their behavior. For example, they need to know what to say if anyone asks them to demonstrate a skill. The best response to such a request would be for the student to say that he or she cannot help but will get someone who has the needed expertise.

Students need some guidance in knowing what they are to observe. For example, the focus might be on the roles of the nurse in the clinic or might be to identify nursing interventions that would be helpful to the clinic clients.

If students are expected to demonstrate skills and assist nurses or physicians, the acceptable skills should be specified. The nurses and physicians in the clinic need to know the limitations on student activities. In order to observe a student, arrange to be present at the initiation of an examination or procedure. This will be less distracting to the student, other health care workers, and the client than will entering a room during some activity.

Home Visits

It is hard to be unobtrusive when the patient, the student, and faculty are sitting in the patient's living room. In the first place, having the student there is an unusual event in the patient's life. At the beginning of the visit, the faculty member should clarify the reason for being there. Some patients will tend to talk to the faculty when they should be talking to the student. Redirect the communication to the student. Find out in advance what the student plans to say to the patient. Help the student to fill in gaps or correct misconceptions before the visit.

Fostering a Positive Climate for Learning

Expectations

One thing that helps to make students feel safe and comfortable in a learning situation is their knowledge of what is expected of them. Try to give students an idea of what observations faculty will be making in the clinical setting. When discussing performance, link comments to specific objectives and course requirements.

There are some aspects of the students' clinical behavior that faculty assume they should know, but their actions show they do not. For example, a student in a community health setting worked with a patient whose son would start crying as soon as he saw anyone in uniform. This had happened the first time the student went to visit the family. The student was given permission to visit the family wearing street clothes.

The faculty assumed she knew this was an exception for that one situation. The student assumed that because it would be complicated to change clothes before or after the visits, she could wear street clothes on all her visits. When the student and one of the staff nurses made a visit together to another family, the staff nurse confronted her about her inappropriate attire. The student told her that the faculty member had approved it, so the nurse approached the faculty and the confusion was rectified.

Assertiveness

One of the expectations for students is for them to become assertive and to take initiative in giving nursing care. Be sure the students understand the limits their initiative can take. When students are assertive, reinforce this behavior. For example, Dan was assigned to a patient whose left leg was in a full leg cast. The woman was in her 50s and had been to physical therapy earlier in the morning. She had not been back on the unit for long before she was scheduled to walk with crutches on the unit. She told the student she was too tired from physical therapy and she wanted to rest for a while before trying crutch walking. When the nurse asked Dan why he did not get the patient up on crutches, he told her what the patient had said. The nurse told him the patient was lazy. Dan pointed out to the nurse that the woman was not accustomed to much physical exertion, she had only been up on crutches once before, and she had had an extensive session in physical therapy. He said he would not label the patient as lazy and he thought it was legitimate for her to wait until later in the morning for more activity.

Even when students make mistakes, such as in the situation just described, try to foster assertiveness while helping them examine and correct the behavior.

Self-Esteem

Whenever one is in a student role, self-esteem is greatly affected by one's learning experiences. In nursing education, many of the young people have been students for virtually their entire lives. Their self-concepts tend to center around being students, and things that happen to them in this role determine their self-esteem. This helps to explain why they can get so passionate about the difference between an A and a B on a test, for example.

In the clinical area, students have their behavior evaluated in a way most of them have never experienced in another situation. This is a much more emotionally laden experience than marking answers on a test or writing a term paper. A lot of what they are evaluated on is close to what constitutes their personalities. For example, the way a student interacts with a patient is partially determined by that student's culture, family, personal experiences, and self-concept. When faculty critique the student's skill, deeply held beliefs and values may be threatened, however unintentionally. Because of this, a student's reactions to the faculty member's remarks may sometimes be perplexing.

An insecure student may treat a comment considered just a suggestion as a mandate. Another comment intended to be funny may hurt a student's feelings. The problem with this is that faculty probably will not realize immediately that such comments had these results.

When students make mistakes, do not heap blame or criticism on them. They are often much harder on themselves. Be sure that students appreciate the impact of errors they make, but also help them to put such incidents in perspective. Students need to know when they are doing well. Let them know this as directly as possible. Rather than simply saying, "You met the objectives," add specific positive comments, such as, "You were so gentle, and it was obvious the patient appreciated it," or "You did that as if you had been doing it all your life," or "Yes, it was a little prolonged, but you explained everything so well, I do not think it bothered the patient."

The clinical faculty is the expert whose role is to make judgments about each student's performance. Part of making those judgments is helping students to reinforce strengths, not just to eliminate weaknesses. Students should end their experience knowing more about nursing but also feeling more confident about themselves as they evolve into professional nurses.

Describe behavior and explain why it is or is not acceptable. Try to avoid putting global labels on students or their behavior. For example, do not say, "You are incompetent." Describe what is wrong and why it is a problem. Please do not ever say, "You are never going to be a good nurse," or words to that effect. In the first place, the faculty could be wrong. Maybe that student will be a fantastic nurse in a different setting. In the second place, such a statement does not offer any room for growth.

Faculty members sometimes get upset with students or undermine students' self-esteem, particularly when situations arise that might reflect on the faculty's clinical ability. A faculty member who worries about being blamed might get defensive and show it by getting angry with the student. This faculty member could also get depressed and not look at how the incident could be used to improve student orientation. Faculty should know that they are not perfect and students are not perfect. As long as we are trying to do all we can to promote safe care, the chances of those mistakes being serious are limited.

Helping Students in Difficulty

Overidentification

Sometimes students have trouble with patients when they overidentify with the patient or the patient's situation. This often happens when the student manifests an extreme behavior such as (1) spending too much time or not enough time with the patient, (2) being too restrictive or too permissive with the patient's behavior, (3) arguing with others about the care the patient is or is not getting, (4) doing too much or too little for the patient, or (5) seeming too confident or too reticent in dealing with the patient.

When signals like these are observed, make it a point to talk with the student. Although the student may start out being defensive, he or she may be able to volunteer the information that helps to explain what is happening. For example, a student working with an alcoholic who reminds her of her father may behave inappropriately. With help, she will be able to begin separating her feelings and responsibilities about one from those about the other.

It is obviously more difficult to work with the student who denies the overidentification. Continue to point out behaviors that are inappropriate and try to help the student see this more objectively. The student will have trouble attaining objectivity, however, while still working with the patient. If the student's problem interferes with what is in the patient's best interest, change the student's assignment.

Blocking

Sometimes a student freezes when it is time to do a new procedure, especially if it is an invasive one. It is fairly common for students to have some anxiety about giving their first injection. A few will become immobilized by the anxiety. One of my students gave me no clues that she was any more nervous than the average student about giving her first injection to a patient. We entered the room, she told the patient what she was there for, and she positioned him properly for an injection in his buttock. She pointed out the correct site to me, swabbed it with alcohol, and removed the cap from the needle. My attention was directed to the man's hip, and I realized nothing else seemed to be happening. I looked back at her to see a wide, unblinking stare. I patted her shoulder and nodded for her to go on, as I pointed at the site and smiled encouragingly. Nothing happened. I gently extracted the syringe from her hand and gave the injection myself. She swabbed the man's skin and rearranged the covers over him. I made sure he was comfortable, and we left the room. She leaned against the wall and looked like she might faint or start crying, so I ushered her into an empty room. We talked about what happened, and I assured her I understood her behavior. She finally said she wanted another chance as soon as possible. One of the staff nurses was about to get an injection for one of her patients, and she let the student draw it up. This time, when we went to the room, the student did fine

Sometimes when students block on giving injections or on some other procedure, they almost have an anxiety attack about it. It is best not to push them too hard because this form of blocking represents a severe form of anxiety. Try to work around that particular skill for a while.

Another kind of student blocking happens when you enter the room to observe. No matter how unthreatening they are, faculty will probably make students nervous when watching their performance. It is part of the nature of the situation. Some of this anxiety diminishes as the students have experiences in which faculty are helpful and supportive to them.

However, some students have a chronic problem with being observed. In these cases, try to do things with them rather than just standing and observing them. Arrange to talk with the student before an observation, and be clear about the purpose.

Fortunately, most students get over blocking anxiety, or they learn to function well, even though they are nervous. If they cannot, and if it is just one student here or there, the faculty is not likely to be the real cause. In severe situations, the students may need outside counseling. Talk to the course coordinator before referring students for counseling on such matters.

If many students seem to become very anxious when observed or block when they are trying to perform, the faculty should reflect on their own behaviors. Be objective. Ask a colleague to observe and help identify what might be causing these reactions. Faculty may unintentionally seem stern and unfriendly, causing even secure students to become disorganized.

Conflicts

If a student has a conflict with a patient, try to figure out what is going on so that, unless the patient demands that the student not continue, the student may be able to continue working with the patient. The staff nurse or faculty member should talk with the patient and the student separately to find out about the conflict. As with most conflicts, sometimes it is the patient's problem, sometimes it is the student's problem, and sometimes it is a combination. Sometime students are slow in doing things. Although some patients accept this, others are not able to tolerate it. Slow students usually need more practice or more support to learn to function faster. However, some patients may be very distressed by this behavior. If it appears that there is any hint of conflict after you have tried to resolve the issues, it may be best for both the patient and student if the student is reassigned to another patient or clinical activity.

If students get into conflicts with staff, assess why this is happening. First, find out both sides of the story by talking to the staff members involved and with the student. Get specific descriptions of behaviors related to the conflict. Try to avoid a direct confrontation between staff and student. Find a private area to have conversations about the conflict with the student and the staff member involved as you try to come to a resolution.

Sometimes a student will be abrasive. Preserve the learning experience for the student and be supportive of the staff. They make it possible for all students to learn. If the student is in the wrong, help the student understand what is wrong but also to assure the staff member you have intervened without unduly embarrassing the student.

Serious conflicts between staff and students are rare. When it does happen, it is sometimes because of a particular staff member who has a history of problems with many students and who openly objects to working with nursing students. Other conflicts occur because of a problem the student is having. For example, some students are judgmental and condescending to the staff. Other students are poorly organized or overly dependent. These students will bother the staff. When confronted, the student is likely to blame the staff rather than accept responsibility.

Sometimes faculty will have conflicts with students. Conflict usually arises because of differing expectations. If the conflict seems to be with only one or two students, it is most likely due to these students as individuals. Have the same expectations for all students and apply grading criteria equitably. Some new faculty members expect too much from their students. Others are so concerned about the welfare of the patients that they convey to the students a lack of trust in them.

Nonclinical Student Difficulties

Student may have difficulties outside the clinical setting that may impact their success. The faculty member needs to have an antenna raised for these types of issues. The student body is changing rapidly. Many of our students are older, more diverse, and often English is not their first language. Our students may have families to support and are working long hours in addition to going to school, may experience adverse family issues, and have poor support systems. They may experience stress, anxiety and role strain. Students with these types of difficulties are at higher risk of failure or of dropping out of the program altogether. Seek an opportunity to have a quiet talk with a student you suspect has any of these difficulties. Discuss the support available on campus for the student, and advise the student to go to student counseling for assistance. Follow up with the student periodically, and document your interactions with the student.

Knowing More Than the Students

Sometimes your students will ask questions you cannot answer. Do not try to fake it. Give them the message that it is okay to still be learning, even when you are a professional.

Do not try to evade a question by merely telling the student to look it up. Suggest that the student and faculty find out the answer together. This shows the student that learning is ongoing. Helping a student to identify sources of knowledge is an important aspect of clinical experiences. Students need to know what they do not know and, what is more important, where to find the information.

Anecdotal Notes

Most faculty members keep a record of the important aspects of students' performance through anecdotal notes. As the name implies, the notes report anecdotal comments about students' progress in the clinical area. Such notes help in day-to-day counseling of students and provide data for evaluation. Make note of accomplishments as well as of learning needs indicated by incidents in the clinical area. Some faculty members like to keep a table with the types of experiences the student has had, for example, type of patient, age range, experience with medication, IVs, communication skills, and so forth. This table can be used when planning future assignments because it makes it easy to identify gaps in the student's experience.

Form

The form is probably the least important aspect of anecdotal records. You can use a PDA, a notebook, or whatever is convenient. Entries are usually explicit and document incidents that support how the student is or is not meeting the objectives. Make sure these are stored in a secure place because they contain student information.

Timeliness

The most important requirement of an anecdotal note is that it be made as close as possible in time to the actual events. It is easy to forget and distort things with the passage of time, so it helps to write down comments as soon as possible.

Content

The content of an anecdotal note should be made up of descriptive observations about the students' behavior. This will help in writing evaluations and can better help the student to understand how conclusions were drawn. Avoid judgmental statements. Table 2.1 shows a sample anecdotal note.

TABLE 2.1   Anecdotal Note

Note on Lisa 8/23/12
Worked w/32 y/o woman, postop 2 days, splenectomy. L. asked pt. when she wanted a shower and planned around it. Found out woman was trying to lose weight and wanted a diet. L. got order for this & informed dietary. Planned for this keeping in mind need for her body to heal. Did not check chart for new orders & was late giving 1st dose of new med. I would not have known this, but she told me herself, as well as how she would avoid this oversight in future.

Access

Anecdotal notes should be treated as confidential documents; although these notes are confidential, the course coordinator or grievance board could request them if there is any question about the student evaluation and final grade.

Evaluating Clinical Performance

Clinical Content

The specific content of what students should accomplish in the clinical area is determined by the objectives. The particular clinical area as well as school policy will determine the way students are evaluated. Some programs have specific expectations with levels of achievement identified, so number or letter grades can be given. Other programs may have certain minimal expectations that all students must achieve, but the grade for clinical is Satisfactory or Unsatisfactory.

The clearer the expectations and their association with the grading system, the less difficult it is to arrive at a grade. There is no way to avoid the fact that evaluating clinical performance is subjective. Objectively written criteria minimize subjectivity. However, even the application of objective criteria is affected by the values of the evaluator. For example, two faculty members might both observe a skill exercised by a student. One might be more flexible about deviations from the usual way the skill is done as long as the student does it safely and ends up with the correct result. The other might think it is important to include every step just as he or she learned it. On the other hand, the stricter faculty member might allow students to be more casual in their interactions with patients than the other member would expect. These differences could lead to different grades. However, the more explicit the criteria and the more agreement there is about expectations and values, the closer two faculty members will be in assigning grades.

With experience, you will become more confident. Develop a grading rubric for each assignment that will help all faculty involved in grading give similar grades. Share the grading rubric with students so the process is transparent.

In some clinical settings, it may be useful to develop a learning contract. This helps to make expectations explicit and makes it clearer that the students determine their grades by their behavior. Chapter 3 describes that process of developing a learning contract.

Professional Behavior

Unlike some content-related behaviors, there are certain professional expectations that are either present or absent. Sometimes it may be difficult to spell out these expectations, which are as significant as any related to safe patient care. Tables 2.2 and 2.3 show lists of behaviors that indicate the presence or absence of values related to professionalism.

Frequently, the area of most concern with students relates to their inability to provide nursing care in a professional way. Even though they make good grades, they seem to lack a real concern or regard for patients. It is legitimate to build these expectations into grading criteria. Specifying such expectations and spelling out that students must consistently demonstrate these behaviors give support if these behaviors must be adhered to in order to pass clinical.

Formative and Summative

Formative evaluation is that process that helps a student to achieve the final objectives. Usually this evaluation is informal, such as telling students on a weekly basis how they have done in the clinical area. At the midpoint of the term, give a slightly more formal evaluation of students' performance so that they know what they have accomplished and what they need to achieve in the remainder of the term. Generally, a grade is not attached to such assessments because they are meant to promote growth. Summative evaluations are done at the end of an experience in order to evaluate the student's ability to meet the terminal objectives. A grade is usually attached to summative evaluations.

Evaluating students on a day-to-day basis is a formative process. Although the clinical practice time may be compressed, students need to be allowed to practice skills and behaviors before they are actually graded on them. Students become intimidated when faculty begins grading behaviors immediately. How can they feel they are really in a learning environment if they are penalized for needing to learn?

Conferences

Preclinical

Faculty members usually have a brief conference with students at the beginning of the clinical day in order to share information, to validate

LE 2.2   Behaviors Implying the Presence of Professional Values

: Placing the patient's welfare first
   ccessible and prompt in answering patient's requests
     ity of activities reflects patient's needs
       ns treatments and procedures; keeps patient well informed
   ₋ responsive and reliable when needs are identified by patients, staff, or
      faculty
   Calls and makes appropriate arrangements if unable to be on time or
      present for clinical

Value: Commitment to nursing and to nursing department policies
   Present and willing to learn; complies voluntarily with rules and policies
      of the nursing department
   Demonstrates enthusiasm for clinical; appears to enjoy nursing
   Looks and acts in a professional manner (i.e., is neat and clean; behaves
      in a professional way)
   Pleasant to staff, peers, and faculty
   Gives appropriate information to other nurses
   Completes charts and records

Value: Cooperation
   Able to disagree diplomatically
   Knows when to stop arguing and start helping
   Takes criticism constructively
   Accepts the roles of others and works in an appropriate capacity in
      response to others
   Deals with stress and frustration without taking it out on others
   Objectively handles conflict with others; tries to see both sides of issues

Value: Intellectual and personal integrity
   Readily admits mistakes and oversights
   Forthright with peers, staff, and faculty
   Selects appropriate response to patients
   Observes safe technique, even when not being supervised
   Accepts responsibility for errors and tries to take appropriate actions
   Statements appear to be based on fact and believable
   Does own work and does not represent the work of others as being
      original
   Respectful of faculty, staff, peers, and patients

TABLE 2.3   Behaviors Implying the Absence of Professional Values

Value: Placing the patient's welfare first
  Unreliable in completion of tasks
  Difficult to find when needed
  Elicits hostility from patients and others
  Displays hostility toward difficult patients
  Justifies doing things just for the experience, without taking patient's
    needs into consideration
  Approach is who is right, not what is right
  Fails to make appropriate arrangements if unable to be on time or
    present for clinical

Value: Commitment to nursing and to nursing department policies
  Chronically tardy or absent
  Skips clinical or other obligations if not supervised
  Passes off assignments or tasks to others when possible
  Chronic malcontent and complainer
  Sloppy
  Gives inappropriate information to others
  Chronically deficient on upkeep of charts and records
  Feels existent policies are irrelevant, unimportant, and nonobligatory

Value: Cooperation
  Argumentative or stubborn
  Sullen or arrogant with faculty, peers, staff, and patients
  Uncommunicative with staff and faculty
  Hostile responses to frustrating situations
  Passive-aggressive behavior when dissatisfied

Value: Intellectual and personal integrity
  Lies or fabricates data when needed to cover up mistakes and oversights
  Fails to use safe technique when not being supervised
  Blames others for own shortcomings
  Provides data without appropriate checks for correctness
  Sneaks away or does not show up if unsupervised
  Represents the work of others as being original
  Disrespectful and rude to faculty, staff, peers, or patients

preparation, or simply to convey information. This conference is usually short, especially if it is prior to the day shift. A preclinical conference can set the stage for the clinical day. The faculty member can review the learning objectives for the day; students can ask questions about their patient assignments; the faculty member can prepare students by going through a reminder checklist ranging from checking the emergency equipment, reviewing patient records and medications, and checking patient armbands. For the novice student, this checklist helps to instill confidence because it gives the student definite activities to perform at the beginning of the clinical day as the student settles into caring for the assigned patient.

Postclinical

It is common for faculty to meet in conference with students after their daily or weekly clinical experience. Determine what will be covered in these conferences; for example, to convey content, such as explicit details of a procedure or to discuss the salient events the students experienced during the clinical period.

Some faculty members expect students to take turns in presenting their patients to the rest of the group. The focus can be on the use of the nursing process or on a specific problem. The conference could be used to review specific activities or objectives and to review how the students accomplished these. Take the opportunity to work with the course faculty in selecting topics that the student has covered in class. It is likely that there is a clinical component of the topic that could be presented and discussed in the clinical setting. One topic that lends itself well to almost any clinical situation is family health history. Students will have learned this topic in the classroom and perhaps learned how to draw a pedigree. In the clinical setting, the students could take a family health history from a patient and draw the related pedigree. The clinical faculty can support classroom learning by reviewing the pedigrees in postclinical conference and have the students discuss aspects of family health history and risk of disease. This helps to bridge the gap between the classroom and clinical setting.

This is also a good opportunity for vicarious learning, such as when a student has had a unique experience to share with the group. Nurse managers or other clinical personnel can be invited.

FINAL WORDS

Supervising students in any clinical area may produce high degrees of anxiety for students and faculty. As faculty gain experience, they become less anxious. Try to make it as positive and growth producing as possible for the student. Set your standards high and your students will reach to achieve them.

FURTHER READING

Adams, V. (2002). Consistent clinical assignment for nursing students compared to multiple placements. *Journal of Nursing Education, 41*(2), 80.

Murphy, J. (2004). Using focused reflection and articulation to promote clinical reassuring: An evidenced based teaching strategy. *Nursing Education Perspectives, 25*(5), 226–236.

Sharif, F., & Masoumi, S. (2005). A qualitative study of nursing student experiences of clinical practice. *BMC Nursing, 4*(6). doi: 10.1186/1472–6955–4-6

Vessey, J. A., & Huss, K. (2002). Using standardized patients in advanced practice nursing education. *Journal of Professional Nursing, 18*(1), 29–35. doi:10.1053/jpnu.2002.30898

Zary, N., Johnson, G., Boberg, J., & Fors, U. G. H. (2006). Development, implementation and pilot evaluation of a Web-based virtual patient case simulation environment—Web-SP. *BMC Medical Education, 6*(10). doi:10.1186/1472–6920–6-10

3

Designing a Learning Contract

A learning contract is one method of planning students' work and determining their success. The student and faculty member work collaboratively to create the learning contract. They identify how the student will achieve specific learning outcomes and a grade for his or her work. The learning contract places the responsibility and control of the learning in the hands of the student. The faculty member begins by specifying the amount and quality of work required for each grade, then the student chooses the grades for which he or she is willing to work. This is helpful in courses with requirements that make grading difficult, as well as in courses that have several clinical sections graded by different instructors. For example, some assignments may be easier to evaluate in terms of the quantity of students' participation if the quality is not easily assessed. A study of a community agency might yield the same basic data for a good or a weak student. However, students have the opportunity to receive higher grades by investing more time in the study, by interviewing a wider variety of staff or clients, or by spending more time in the agency.

Contract grading makes it clear that the performance of the student is directly connected to the grade, and the student can choose how much effort he or she is willing to put into a given course or assignment. This method is often used with clinical grading, but it is also useful with other complex assignments. The option of choosing how much effort to expend gives the student more autonomy in meeting the goals of clinical practice or an assignment.

Some of the advantages of using contracts are that students feel less competitive with each another. If they all contract for an A and achieve all the work necessary, they can all earn an A. In addition, contracts make expectations explicit, so students feel there is more objectivity on the part of faculty. Some students also feel a greater sense of responsibility for their learning, and faculty may find that contract learning facilitates learning among an increasingly diverse student population. Many students have experienced some exposure to contract grading and are comfortable using contracts. A disadvantage frequently cited by faculty and students is that contracts seem to place more emphasis on quantity than on quality. However, this can be rectified by building in qualitative criteria along with other contract elements. These criteria may include evidence of teamwork and collaboration in the clinical situation. For a course assignment, qualitative criteria could include evidence of depth of understanding of a topic or evidence of having read a wide range of supplemental sources.

GOALS

The principal goal of using contracts in evaluating and grading students is to increase student autonomy and control. In addition, contract learning reinforces active, independent learning and assists a student to develop self-directed learning skills and ultimately fosters lifelong learning. Contract learning assists the student to integrate theory into practice by utilizing a variety of individualized clinical learning strategies. Contract grading also promotes objectivity in evaluation.

TOOLS

Objectives

The objectives for the clinical experience or assignment determine the format of the contract. Regardless of the grade for which the student contracts, each student has to meet every objective to some extent. The contract will specify how that will be done for each grade.

Format

Table 3.1 outlines the principal components of the contract material. The example is from the clinical component of a course in community health nursing.

Introduction

Start with an introduction that explains the use of the contract. This will be a new experience for many students. They need a good understanding of what will be involved.

Objectives

List the objectives that will be met with the contract. It is important for students to see connections between contract specifications and the objectives.

Performance Requirements

For each objective, list the performance requirements for each grade level. Usually, all students are expected to meet the basic performance standards. As they work to achieve higher grades, additional work may be expected for each increment. In addition, students working toward higher grades may be expected to meet higher qualitative standards of practice when they complete the basic requirements.

TABLE 3.1   Contract Requirements for Community Health Clinical Experience

---

Introduction: The purpose of the contract is to permit you (the student) to determine the amount and quality of work for the experience. After reading the requirements for each grade, complete the contract form and be prepared to discuss it with your instructor at the set time.

Objectives: At the end of this clinical experience, you will be able to:

1. Plan and carry out visits to clients in their homes
2. Describe and analyze interpersonal interactions with clients
3. Develop and maintain ongoing nursing care plans for clients in the community
4. Plan and implement effective teaching strategies with community clients
5. Make appropriate referrals for community clients
6. Describe and compare the roles of nurses in the community

Performance Requirements:

Grade of C

1. Follow one client or family
   Make weekly home visits

(continued)

TABLE 3.1   *(continued)*

___

Maintain appropriate records at the agency
Maintain an ongoing nursing care plan
Have written objectives for each visit
Maintain drug cards as needed
Make appropriate referrals as needed

2. Submit your care plan to the instructor each week
3. Meet with the instructor weekly to discuss the progress of work with your client
4. Attend and participate in weekly group conference with instructor and peers
5. Attend clinics and other activities as scheduled once a week
6. Complete one process recording that meets minimum requirements as specified in the course syllabus
7. Complete one teaching project that meets minimum requirements
8. Using contract criteria, complete weekly self-evaluations and a summative evaluation at the end of the term

Grade of B

1. Meet all the requirements for a grade of C except that the nursing care plan, teaching plan, and process recording must meet B-level criteria as specified in the course syllabus
2. Follow one additional client or family, meeting the same expectations as with the first
3. Read three journal articles on the clinical application of community theory and prepare bibliography cards on the articles

Grade of A

1. Meet all the requirements for a grade of C except that the nursing care plan, teaching plan, and process recording must meet A-level criteria as specified in the course syllabus
2. Follow one additional client or family, meeting the same expectations as with the first
3. Read three journal articles on the clinical application of community theory and prepare bibliography cards on the articles
4. Complete a special focus process recording (PR) with specific learning objectives agreed upon with the clinical instructor. The PR must reflect creativity and meet the criteria for the A level
5. Write a brief paper (three to four typed pages) focusing on the counseling role of the nurse; use at least two references and include one or more examples from your own clinical experience

Contract Form

The final component is the actual contract to be signed by each student and the faculty member, specifying the intended grade. The contract form should include a section for reviewing and renegotiating at a given point. Table 3.2 shows a contract form corresponding with the material in Table 3.1.

Checklist

Another item that may be helpful is a checklist to initial as a student satisfies each requirement. Space can be incorporated for evaluative comments. At the end of the semester, this provides the basis for the evaluation, and a copy can be filed. An example of a checklist is shown in Table 3.3.

TABLE 3.2   Contract Form

Community Health Clinical Student Contract

This form is to be signed by the student and the faculty member by the end of the first clinical week. After reading the performance requirements, you will indicate the grade you will work toward. If you do not satisfy all the requirements for the contracted grade, you will receive the grade for which you have met requirements.

At any time during the term, you may ask to renegotiate. If you want to change to a higher grade, sufficient time must remain for you to achieve it. If you want to change to a lower grade, any commitments to clients must be completed.

I, _____, have read the performance requirements for the community health clinical experience and will work for a grade of _____.

_____   _____
Student   Clinical instructor

I wish to change the original terms. As of this date, I will work for a grade of _____.

_____   _____
Student   Clinical instructor

TABLE 3.3   Contract Checklist

Student_____ Term_____

Contracted grade_____

Criteria for all clinical activities will be the level described in the course syllabus as determined by the contracted grade.

Requirements for all grades:

1. Client/family visits
    Weeks   1   2   3   4
    Visited weekly
    Record entries
    Care plan in
    Objectives
    Drug cards
    Referrals
2. Meet with instructor
3. Group conferences
4. Clinics
5. PR turned in
6. Teaching project
7. Self-evaluations

Additional requirements for B and A:

1. Second client/family
    Weeks   1   2   3   4
    Visited weekly
    Record entries
    Care plan in
    Objectives
    Drug cards
    Referrals
2. Summary of selected journal articles   No. 1   No. 2   No. 3

Additional requirements for A:

1. Special PR
2. Clinical paper

Comments:

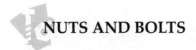

NUTS AND BOLTS

Deadlines

Set deadlines for each activity. Students who want extensions may negotiate for new deadlines. Be aware that negotiations may lead to other consequences because the student may be unable to progress until he or she has achieved the learning outcomes and received a grade in this course.

Validation

Students are responsible for requesting faculty to validate that contract requirements have been met. This is especially important in the clinical setting where many of the requirements may involve psychomotor skills.

When students are ready to demonstrate competence with a required skill, they should find the faculty member and request supervision for this purpose. The student should carry a copy of the checklist so that the faculty member can sign it once the student is competent.

In the clinical and classroom settings, the checklist affords a good guide to help the students stay on top of their responsibilities. In addition to using the checklist, make anecdotal notes to support decisions about the quality of the student's performance.

Criteria

Specify the criteria used to give different letter grades for certain assignments. This helps to demonstrate that the contract is not dependent only on quantity for achieving higher grades. Table 3.4 shows some criteria that could be used to differentiate among the levels when evaluating a teaching plan.

For some activities, simply require the student to complete the work, but do not evaluate it using the criteria. An example would be the observations made in clinics as part of the community health clinical activities.

Giving a Numerical Grade

With most assignments, use a numerical grade as well as a letter grade to be averaged with other components of a course grade. A student

TABLE 3.4   Grade-Level Criteria for Teaching Plan

C Level	B Level	A Level
Assessment		
Obvious data identified	Obvious and subtle data identified	Obvious and subtle data identified
Uses readily available references	Uses additional references	Uses additional references
Nursing diagnosis is obvious	Nursing diagnosis is obvious	Nursing diagnosis is subtle
Planning		
States obvious behavioral objectives that can be measured	All obvious behavioral objectives stated clearly and are measurable	All obvious and some subtle objectives stated clearly and are measurable
Implementation		
Obvious teaching methods with limited skill and preparation used correctly	Teaching methods with moderate preparation and limited skill used correctly	Teaching methods with extensive preparation and moderate skill used correctly
Obvious content is identified	All applicable content is identified	All applicable content is identified
Rationale for methods and content are described and documented by assigned texts	Rationale for methods and content are described and documented by 1 or 2 resources in addition to text	Rationale for methods and content are described and documented by more than 2 resources in addition to texts
Evaluation		
Methods and content are evaluated	Methods and content are evaluated as to effectiveness and appropriateness	Methods and content are evaluated as to effectiveness and appropriateness with discussion of future use

(continued)

TABLE 3.4   *(continued)*

C Level	B Level	A Level
	Evaluation	
Client's ability to meet each behavioral objective is described	Client's ability to meet each behavioral objective is described	Client's ability to meet each behavioral objective is evaluated in a creative way

Note. Adapted from Schoolcraft and Delaney (1982).

may consistently meet the expectations for the contracted letter grade and perhaps even do as well as the next-higher letter on some things. Give the student the highest number in the range for the letter grade. This avoids subjectivity because the grade is clearly linked to achievement of the objectives.

Another student might barely meet the qualitative criteria and may take a long time to start demonstrating skills consistently at the contracted grade level. That student might receive a lower grade in the range. One thing to remember is that a grade of 100 for an A does not mean the student is perfect. It merely means the student consistently accomplished the requirements set for an A for that course.

If the clinical portion of the course receives a letter grade, regardless of the means of reaching it, some students will try to manipulate faculty to give them a few more points. This is especially true if a few points may raise their course grades to a higher letter. Suddenly, someone who could not find the time to look up one extra reference for a teaching plan will invest an hour in trying to get two more points for the clinical grade (see Table 3.4).

Using the Contract

Many students will determine for themselves that they do not want to do the work required for a grade of A. Some students have objected to the contract because they felt they might have gotten higher grades if the requirements had not been so specific.

On the other hand, try to talk students into trying for higher grades when they feel insecure in their abilities. After a few days in clinical, if the student does better than the contracted grade requires, encourage that student to consider doing the additional work. This builds self-confidence and a positive learning outcome. Some students will strive to achieve the higher grade to prove to themselves and the faculty member that they can excel.

Try to give students as much time as reasonable to accomplish the grades they choose. For example, a student contracting for an A may be a slow starter. Give the student as much time as possible to get in the groove. If it becomes apparent that the student cannot handle the expectations for the grade they contracted for, suggest developing a contract for a lower grade.

Additional Applications for Learning Contracts

Learning Contracts to Improve Academic or Clinical Performance

Learning contracts can be used as tools to help students who are not meeting academic and/or clinical course objectives. The contract in this case identifies areas of concern in student performance related to the failure of the student to meet the objectives. In the clinical arena, learning contracts may be created for students who do not meet clinical learning objectives or where clinical performance puts patients' safety at risk. Students can learn from their mistakes through the use of learning contracts. In these situations, the learning outcomes may be linked to clinical performance and patient safety. The student and the faculty member will identify the resources or activities the student needs to use to meet the learning contract objectives. Outcomes that identify how the student is expected to meet the objectives within a specified time are included. The student needs to be aware that consistent successful performance of the outcomes is required to meet the objectives and to pass the course. Once the contract has been written and discussed with the student, both the student and the faculty member should date and sign the contract. The student should be given a copy of the contract. Frequent meetings to provide feedback, perhaps weekly, should be planned as the student works toward meeting the objectives.

Learning Contracts With Diverse Adult Learners

RN-to-BSN students enter nursing programs with a variety of backgrounds and experiences. Some RN-to-BSN students may have little clinical nursing experience while others may have decades of experience. Learning contracts provide an opportunity for students with diverse practice backgrounds to individualize their educational process and progress. Students choose the most effective learning strategies to meet the course objectives. The responsibility for learning shifts from the faculty member to the student throughout the process. Initially, the faculty member assists the student to identify his or her learning needs. Secondly, the faculty member provides the student with instructions on how to write learning objectives. Next, the student will need to indentify learning resources and activities to meet the identified objectives. The final portion of the contract involves identifying the evidence the student will demonstrate to meet the learning objectives and the grade for the assignments. This type of learning contract works well with the adult learner returning to education following clinical work experience.

FINAL WORDS

Learning contracts offer a variety ways of giving the student more independence in the clinical area. Contracts help to defuse some of the anxiety that students experience when the faculty member observes them because the students can determine when they are ready to be evaluated. They know in advance which criteria they have to meet. It does not remove all the difficulties of grading, but it can be a helpful tool.

FURTHER READING

Billings, D. M., & Halstead, J. A. (2009). *Teaching in nursing: A guide for faculty.* St Louis, MO: Saunders.

Chan, S. W., & Wai-tong, C. (2000). Implementing contract learning in a clinical context. *Journal of Advanced Nursing, 31*(2), 298–305.

Chien, W., & Chan, S.W-t. (2002). The use of learning contracts in the mental health nursing clinical placement: An action research. *International Journal of Nursing Studies, 39,* 685–694.

Gregory, D., Guse, L., Davidson, D., Davis, P., & Russel, C. K. (2009). What clinical learning contracts reveal about nursing education and safety. *Canadian Nurse, 10,* 20–25.

Schoolcraft, V., & Delaney, C. (1982). Contract grading in clinical evaluation. *Journal of Nursing Education, 21,* 6–14.

Waddell, D. L., & Stephens, S. (2000). Use of learning contract in a RN-to-BSN leadership course. *The Journal of Continuing Education in Nursing, 31*(4), 179–184.

4

Teaching Students to Work in Groups

Nurses and other health care providers work in teams, so it makes sense that faculty provide nursing students with opportunities to accomplish learning goals by working together. Small-group learning actively engages both students and faculty. It promotes interpersonal communication as well as critical reasoning and problem solving—necessary skills for nursing students entering an ever-changing health care environment.

Although some faculty members give students guidance in working together, many do not. Faculty often expects students to know how to work in groups without considering where they are supposed to acquire the necessary skills. They need to have reasonable expectations of students when creating small-group assignments. When expectations are not appropriate, students may become so bogged down in the group process that they are unable to meet the learning objectives of the activity. Getting the students to work successfully in groups may be harder than you think, especially when they have not done it before. If students have not been exposed to concepts about effective group work, faculty should plan to teach this skill. Good group dynamics are key to successful group work. As a first step you may create opportunities for students to get to know each other and to develop trust with each other within the learning environment. The introduction of some icebreaker activities at the beginning of a course can set the stage for good group dynamics. Teaching students some best practices, such as developing a set of rules for communication and decision making within the group, how to deal with conflict, and communicating with the faculty will help the group work to go smoothly.

GOALS

The primary goal of teaching the dynamics of group functioning is to promote effective group work. A secondary goal is to foster student appreciation for learning and working in groups.

APPROACHES TO GROUP LEARNING

Problem-based learning (PBL) is a collaborative learning approach utilizing case studies to facilitate problem solving; it is typically done in small groups with a faculty facilitator. The advantages of this type of learning is that it promotes learning new concepts, helps identify student learning needs, and fosters critical reasoning in a safe, simulated case experience. The disadvantage is that it is resource intense—it requires several faculty members acting as facilitators.

Team-based learning (TBL) is a collaborative learning approach in which instruction modules involve a three-step cycle (preclass preparation, readiness assurance, and application-focused activity). With this approach there are small student groups but only one faculty facilitator for all the groups in the class with as many as 200 students in total. One advantage of this learning approach is that the student groups remain the same throughout the course. Consistent groups and sequential learning modules facilitate team development. Other advantages are the same as those noted in PBL. As in PBL, the disadvantages include the time commitment required by faculty.

INTERPROFESSIONAL GROUPS

The ability to work in groups extends beyond the classroom. Nurses need to communicate and collaborate with members of the health care team in order to provide holistic, patient-centered care. In an effort to promote quality care and patient safety, faculty are called on to embrace facilitation of both intra- and interprofessional groups learning.

National initiatives such as the Institute of Medicine and the Quality and Safety in Education for Nurses (QSEN) program have placed a value on interprofessional teams as a key component in patient-centered care. Interprofessional learning and practice is most successful when competencies such as communication, one's own professional role, knowledge of the professional role of others, and conflict resolution are addressed by students and faculty members. Faculty can provide students with simulations or exercises that explore these competencies. Nursing and medical students have said they really do not know what their counterparts can do or how they learn.

Health professionals and educators should collaborate on experiential learning activities and provide students the opportunity to practice in interprofessional teams. Examples include an interprofessional education experience with group learning activities used to address the role that communication and teamwork play in patient safety. Service learning is another suitable opportunity to facilitate interprofessional learning.

TOOLS

Guidelines for Effective Group Work

Structure

Set some of the structural aspects, such as the number of students who will work in each group, how the group membership will be determined, and the focus of their work together. Three or four students would be an optimal number. If part of the purpose of having students work together is to focus on group process, they need more than two in a group. If more than five students in a group, the workload may be spread too thin, or some students may not participate equitably.

Assign students to the group membership, or allow students to select their own partners. If the group work is to take place during class time, assign people to groups in order to help them get to know and work with people other than their friends. If the group work is going to take several hours out of class, let students pick their own partners to make it easier for them to arrange group meetings. Another option for an online class is to assign students to groups and set up their groups within WebCT or Blackboard. You are able to set up the groups so that each group works individually and does not have access to the work of other groups.

Establish the focus when you describe the assignment and set the objectives. Students may focus on both content and process, in which case you must set objectives for both. For example, in a pediatric course, some of the objectives focused on their group process. A written paper addressed the content of the study. They also dealt with their process by submitting a written statement of their respective responsibilities, their timeframe for the group work, a discussion of their work together when they met with the faculty member, and a summary of their group work that was submitted with the final paper. It is often beneficial to have students prepare and present a brief overview of their group work to the whole class and to spend time in class discussion. This class presentation can be a face to face in class or use Internet-supported technology for distant students.

Other structural aspects have to be worked out by each group. Provide them with some guidance in doing this. A timetable like the one in Table 4.1 may help the students to accomplish their work. They could use this timetable as it is or develop a more detailed one that would specify the agenda for each meeting (see Table 4.1). Students may plan to meet face-to-face, use a chat-room forum supported by their academic institution's computer technology such as WebCT, Blackboard, Second Life, or any of the emerging technologies available for group meetings. Online document-sharing tools are useful for reviewing and collating the work of the individual group members.

Process

In addition to specifying the expectations for their performance in the group, give the students some help in working together. Successful groups engage, respect, and value all group members. Suggestions and feedback are encouraged; teaching students ways to give feedback is important. Include topics such as the importance of nonverbal language, use of neutral stance and neutral language, and timeliness of feedback. Make sure students understand that the purpose of constructive feedback is to help them improve. Feedback should be descriptive and directed to the action not the person. When giving feedback, students should use the words *I* and *me*. During the feedback session, students should state the facts with supporting evidence

TABLE 4.1   Timetable for Group Work

First Meeting

1. Identify focus (e.g., assignment or problem)
2. Discuss approach and distribute work
   Individual responsibilities
   Group responsibilities
3. Establish a schedule and deadlines
4. Plan for presentation of report
   Oral: Set time to assign parts and plan format
   Written: Arrange for typing, proofing, and submitting document

Other Meetings

1. Review work done by individuals
2. Do group work
3. Assess progress in meeting deadlines
4. Identify problems and work on solutions

Last Meeting

1. Assemble individual work and review as a group
2. Complete group work
3. Make final arrangements for presentation of report

and the effect it had on them, and then give some recommendations. This type of format gives structure to the feedback session and avoids any anger or uncivil behaviors. In addition, it models best practices for giving feedback that can be used in any setting or situation. Giving students printed guidelines or ground rules is helpful, especially when engaging them in a simulation to practice these behaviors. Table 4.2 lists some guidelines.

Simulations

A simulation is a structured experience allowing students the opportunity to practice skills prior to using them in real-world situations. Simulations may be used to help students learn group skills in general, or they may help students to practice before undertaking a specific group project. Simulations of problem-solving and creative-thinking situations and other kinds of group exercises can be helpful in conveying useful theory as well as providing an opportunity for application. For example, the following question could be considered for each small

TABLE 4.2   Effective and Creative Group Work

Promoting Effective Thinking

1. Make expectations explicit
2. Take risks and persevere
3. Expand perceptions
4. Challenge assumptions
5. Suspend judgment
6. Foster self-esteem
7. Be patient
8. Tolerate ambiguity and chaos

Fostering a Supportive Group

1. All the group members should have the right to protect their self-image
2. Aggression in the group should be directed toward the problem, not toward group members
3. Effective group work results in everyone winning

Brainstorming Ground Rules

1. No criticism of ideas is allowed during the brainstorming phase
2. Far-out ideas are encouraged, because they may trigger other, more practical ideas from someone else
3. Quantity of ideas is more important than quality

group, using the guidelines in Table 4.2: "How can you find out, in an unobtrusive way, what the people in a given community see as their highest health concern?"

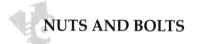

NUTS AND BOLTS

Supervision of Group Assignments

When supervising group assignments, the main challenge is deciding on the ideal amount of faculty involvement. Each group assignment will require different levels of supervision, depending upon the group dynamics, the experience of the students with group work, and the assignment itself. Build in some ongoing contact with groups as they work through a complex assignment. If students are having trouble with either the content or the group process, faculty can help them before they get completely lost. With undergraduates it is a good idea to set up specific meeting times. Early in the group process there may be disagreements and conflicts. This may occur for a number of reasons, such as the students have not worked together in a group before, there is uncertainty related to the task, and the roles of the group members may not be defined. Students may feel unable to make decisions in their group. Meetings with the faculty member may resolve some of these issues, but remember, your role is to facilitate, not take over the group work. One useful strategy for helping the group to work together is providing additional resources on group dynamics along with spending time problem solving with them.

If there are group members who are not doing their share, the other members may be taking on extra work rather than dealing with an unpleasant confrontation. Faculty members fail to deal with such problems within their own ranks, yet they penalize students for not handling these incidents directly.

Try to help students identify their own problems. If they cannot, point it out. Set limits and inform students who are not pulling their own weight. A lower grade might be warranted. In your grading rubric, there may be a section for the group to grade their own group overall as well as the opportunity to grade each of their group colleagues. The faculty member may sum and average the individual grades for each student and include this in their grading score. From experience, this score should reflect at least 10% of the total grade so that it is meaningful, and if the student receives a poor grade from the other students, it could decrease that student's grade by a full letter grade. This gives the student some responsibility for their behavior within the group. The following situation illustrates the complexities of dealing with a problem student.

One student did not show up for the planned meetings with the rest of the group. When other members of the group brought this up in a meeting, the student in question began to give excuses about why she did not come and why she did not contact the others. They reported reasonable efforts to contact her, including trying to talk to her in class. When any of them approached her, she always had a reason she could not talk about. The faculty member told her that if she did not figure out some way to meet with the group and do her share of the work, she would have a failing grade for the assignment. She got angry and insisted on being allowed to do the assignment herself. The student was told that it was meant as a group assignment and it seemed unlikely that she could manage it on her own. She finally agreed to work on the part she had originally been assigned. When the group submitted their paper, the faculty met with them and asked each in turn to describe what she did. In addition, each student in the group was asked to assign a grade for each of the students in their group. The one who had the problems with participating had clearly done less than the others, had given her part to the others late, and had not read the rest of the paper. She did not earn the same grade as the others and was given a grade based only on the quality of her work.

Using Simulations or Exercises

Simulations or exercises should relate to the learning goals for students as well as to the faculty's level of expertise in facilitating group work. The following selection criteria can help faculty members who have little background in facilitating groups:

Criteria

The exercise achieves the identified goals.

The exercise fits with earlier and later exercises.

Materials required can be easily obtained or are easy to construct.

Facilitation of the exercise can be described in clearly written steps.

The exercise is not likely to be emotionally distressing to the participants.

The exercise is interesting and fun to do.

The exercise has perceived value to the participants.

The exercise is easy to facilitate.

Designing a Simulation or Exercise

To design and simulation or exercise, start by writing out the steps in the exercise. Try it out on a group of your colleagues or friends before trying it with students. This will establish some important factors: the actual time involved to complete the exercise, the clarity of the instructions, and the suitability of the exercise to accomplish the goals.

There are many concepts that can be explored with students by using group activities. An experiential approach often has more impact than simply telling students about the concept. Activities that encourage students to actively listen, share information, and weigh the contributions of other group members help create new learning. Some topics to consider for exercises are:

Group task and group maintenance roles assumed by group members

Goal setting

Effective group planning

Role exploration and clarification

Thinking creatively (brainstorming)

Group problem solving

Effect of synergy in group problem solving

Benefits of two-way communication as contrasted with one-way communication

Distortions that occur when rumors are spread

Assertive or apathetic behavior in groups

Effective group planning

Outcomes of competition and cooperation

In addition, see Table 4.3 for an example of a group exercise guide.

TABLE 4.3   Guide for a Group Exercise[a]

Creative Thinking/Brainstorming

GOALS:

1. To identify aspects of creativity
2. To practice brainstorming

TIME REQUIRED: 1 to 1-1/2 hours

MATERIALS:

1. Guidelines for effective and creative group work
2. Paper and writing instrument for each participant

PROCESS:

1. Give everyone an opportunity to read the guidelines.
2. Discuss the guidelines and clarify as needed.

(continued)

TABLE 4.3 *(continued)*

3. Individually, the participants are to write down as many unusual uses as they can for one standard building brick (8.5″ x 4″ x 2.5″); allow 10 minutes. Emphasize this is to be done individually. One brick is all they are focusing on. They should avoid conventional uses for bricks.
4. After their lists are made, tell them not to change or add to their lists, but they may refer to their lists during the group discussion.
5. As a group, they will brainstorm to produce unusual uses for the brick using the information included in the guidelines; allow 20 minutes. Someone should list ideas on the board or flip chart. They may volunteer uses from their own lists. They should keep trying to produce ideas for the entire time.
6. At the end of the brainstorming session, the participants will evaluate their own lists for the following aspects of creativity:
   Fluency: The total number of different uses
   Flexibility: The number of different kinds of uses
   Originality: Everyone will read the uses they have listed; as a use is named, anyone who has the same use must cross it off, including the person who read it; continue around the group until each list contains uses no one else thought of; these uses are then totaled.
7. Figure the same three scores for the group list
   Fluency: Total uses
   Flexibility: Total different kinds of uses
   Originality: Total uses not on any individual lists that were generated during brainstorming
8. Ask participants to share their scores; emphasize that this is a crude measure of creativity.
9. Discuss the participants' responses to using brainstorming techniques.

[a]Victoria Schoolcraft developed this exercise while on the faculty of the University of Oklahoma College of Nursing.

TABLE 4.4 Interpersonal Skills Rubric (Group Process)

Instructions: Must be completed at the conclusion of the group project assignment. Each student must evaluate self-behaviors that helped the group to function effectively, using the outcomes statements and the rating scale provided. Each student should complete the specific questions regarding observations made while functioning within the group process.

Outcomes statements:

1. Keeps the group on task
2. Supports/praises the efforts of others

(continued)

TABLE 4.4   *(continued)*

  3. Encourages participation
  4. Validates understanding of others/self
Rating Scale: 2 = Outstanding
                      1 = Demonstration of the four interpersonal skills
                      0 = No demonstration of the four interpersonal skills
Score: _____ (Assigned by instructor)

Complete the following questions, utilizing observations/thoughts assessing the group process during the group project assignments:

  1. Who emerged as group leader?
  2. Was the person appointed or assumed the leadership role?
  3. When in the process did the leader emerge?
  4. Was there a power struggle within the group?
  5. Who was/were the listener(s) and thinker(s) within the group?
  6. Who was the one who most attempted to redirect/keep the group on task, and what did you perceive to be the motivation for the person's doing so?
  7. Was there someone most apt to steer the group off topic? How and why do you think it happened?
  8. Identify at least one positive and one negative interaction (regarding the process, not the topic) you learned during the group process.
  9. In your assessment of the group, do you feel each member equally shared the assignment? If not, give specifics of the situation.

FINAL WORDS

After a group exercise or project is completed, the process may be evaluated using a rubric such as the one in Table 4.4. Identifying effective behaviors, as well as barriers, may provide growth as an individual and as a member of a team.

FURTHER READING

Clark, M., Nguyen, H., Bray, C., & Levine, R. (2008). Team-based learning in an undergraduate nursing course. *Journal of Nursing Education, 47*(3), 111–117.

Gallagher, P. (2009). Collaborative essay testing: Group work that counts. *International Journal of Nursing Education Scholarship, 6*(1), Art. 37.

MacDonald, M., Bally, J., Ferguson, L., Murray, B., Fowler-Kerry, S., & Anonsen, J. (2010). Knowledge of the professional role of others: A key interprofessional competency. *Nurse Education in Practice, 10,* 238–242.

Mennenga, H., & Smyer, T. (2010). A model for easily incorporating team-based learning into nursing education. *International Journal of Nursing Education Scholarship, 7*(1), Art. 4.

Morris, D., & Turnbull, P. (2004). Issues and innovations in nursing education. *Journal of Advanced Nursing, 45*(2), 136–145.

Parmelee, D., & Michaelsen, L. (2010). Twelve tips for doing effective team-based learning (TBL). *Medical Teacher, 32,* 118–122.

Posey, L., & Pintz, C. (2006). Online teaching strategies to improve collaboration among nursing students. *Nurse Education Today, 26*(8), 680–687. doi:10.1016/j.nedt.2006.07.015

Rauen, C. A. (2004). Simulation as a teaching strategy for nursing education and orientation in cardiac surgery. *Critical Care Nurse, 24*(3), 46–51.

Rieck, S., & Crouch, L. (2007). Connectiveness and civility in online learning. *Nurse Education in Practice, 7*(6), 425–432. doi:10.1016/j.nepr.2007.06.006

Thompson, S., & Tilden, V. (2009). Embracing quality and safety education for the 21st century: Building interprofessional education. *Journal of Nursing Education, 48*(12), 698–701.

Web Sites of Interest

Institute for Healthcare Improvement: http://www.ihi.org
Quality and Safety Education for Nurses: http://www.qsen.org
Team-Based Learning Collaborative: http://teambasedlearning.org

5

Planning to Give a Lecture

The lecture is an efficient way of imparting knowledge to students, but is it an effective learning strategy? It has been said that a lecture is a way of getting what is in the faculty member's notes into the students' notes without the information necessarily passing through the minds of any of them. Keep this notion in mind as you prepare.

As much as everyone seems to complain about lectures, it is amazing that they persist. Emma hates giving lectures and will do anything to avoid it, Jim accumulates lectures as status symbols, and Helen seems convinced the students must hear each pearl of wisdom from her own lips in order to really know the material.

Many nursing faculty members give lectures because they are relatively easy to prepare. In some academic settings, the number of lectures may contribute to fulfilling a workload commitment, or lectures may help to convey to others an idea of the expertise of faculty members. Finally, there are probably some students who will not learn material unless they hear it from the faculty. Given this range of beliefs, ask the following questions before starting.

"Why am I getting ready to give a lecture?"

The most appropriate answer to any question about teaching methodology should be, "Because this is the most effective way to convey this material to students." If that criterion is not met by a lecture, think about some other options. Maybe a panel of nurses or patients would convey what you want the students to know. Perhaps the reading assignment is sufficient. Maybe a demonstration or observational experience is more appropriate for this topic.

"How do I feel about giving lectures?"

Being nervous will detract from your presentation. A speech course or other endeavor to learn more about public speaking will help overcome nervousness. Maybe the reason for the discomfort relates to the first question—perhaps a lecture is not the best method to use.

"Am I able to give an effective lecture?"

Educators frequently have not considered whether they are effective at lecturing. This leads to many frightening hours for individuals who really do not like to speak to groups and to many boring hours for those who are required to listen. Someone may be an excellent faculty member in other aspects of the faculty appointment and yet be unable to lecture effectively. However, lecturing seems to be an activity faculty members are expected to perform. Diagnose difficulties and start to remedy them immediately.

GOALS

A lecture should offer a summary of important, up-to-date material that is unavailable to students in other forms; provide for clarification of key concepts; and emphasize important content. Ideally, a lecture should not duplicate information from required readings and other resources. A lecturer should repeat things from other sources only for emphasis or explanation. A lecture should stimulate students while developing and expanding their interest and knowledge of the topic. It can also be used to challenge ideas of the students.

TOOLS

Knowledge

Up-to-date knowledge of the content area is vital for a good lecture. Perhaps the biggest shortcomings of ineffective lectures are a lack of pertinent new information and the presentation of information that is too complex for the recipients. If a faculty member lacks knowledge, it may result in a rehash of the assigned readings or a delivery of a superficial review of the content. On the other hand, if a faculty member is an expert on the content or has just finished graduate courses in the field, he or she may tend to teach the content in greater depth or breadth than is required. Information of the student's knowledge is important also. Where does this lecture fit in the program of study? Does the lecture build on knowledge presented in previous courses? It is new knowledge being presented in a single lecture? Answers to these questions will help you to focus your knowledge of the content area to the students' needs.

Objectives

Beforehand, decide what students should know after they have listened to the lecture. Identify what is really important for them to learn and to retain. Students will take away three to five key points from a lecture, so avoid having too many objectives. This will focus the objectives you set. Start by making a list of the concepts that need to be covered. Then decide what students need to know about these ideas. For example, do they need only to know definitions, or should they be able to apply the concepts? This will help determine the correct verbs to use in the objectives.

The objectives should be on a cognitive, psychomotor, or affective level appropriate to the course and the students. Content related to the acquisition and application of knowledge should have objectives in the cognitive realm (knowledge, comprehension, application, analysis, synthesis, and evaluation). Learning related to values, attitudes, appreciation, and personal adjustments calls for objectives in the affective realm (receiving or attending, responding, valuing, conceptualization of a value, organization of a value system, and characterization by a value or value complex). The psychomotor realm pertains to specific motor abilities.

If the course is on a lower level, the objectives should be more basic, such as *define, identify, describe, list,* and so on. More advanced courses would require higher levels of objectives, such as *analyze* and *evaluate.*

Outline

Start organizing the lecture by sketching out the material to be covered in order to help the students meet the objectives. If they should be able to define a certain term, define it for them. If they are supposed to be able to analyze a certain kind of situation, tell them what is important in the situation and how they are supposed to be able to analyze it. If they need to be able to demonstrate a skill, tell them how it should be done, show them how to do it, and offer them the opportunity to practice it. Plan the outline in a logical manner.

Content

After the outline is complete, begin to flesh out the content. Make sure the content flows in a logical order related to the objectives. That would seem obvious, but it is astonishing how frequently lecturers meander about, covering their content without attending to the logical order required to make sense of it. Do not try to cover too much content. The introduction is important as it sets the stage for your lecture. Share the objectives with the class, let them know if you invite questions during the lecture or wish to have questions at the end.

Even though the phrase "a picture is worth a thousand words" applies literally to visual pictures, use word pictures to enhance your content. Include illustrative anecdotes from the clinical area or other aspects of life that will help to clarify and emphasize important points. Be sure to include clinical and other practical examples in notes so that important points will not be forgotten. When organizing notes, include a margin on the right-hand side of the screen that you can use to put cues for, say, time checks (e.g., "should be 15 minutes into lecture"), asking students questions, or including an interactive teaching strategy. These notes to oneself will keep you on track during the lecture. Time passes quickly, and it is easy to run out of time and not have covered the objectives.

Avoid the temptation to spoon-feed students. In addition, students who are given specific information that will be on a test tend to pay attention only to the tested points and ignore learning concepts or nontested items.

The way in which you present your content may be determined by the size of the group or the location of the presentation. Presenting to a small group versus a full auditorium will make a difference in what you include in the content. In addition, the environment in which you are presenting, the set-up of the classroom, and the ability for students to interact may also affect the how you plan to present the content.

Notes

Some faculty members type their complete lectures or use the print outline view or the notes view from PowerPoint or other such programs. Typing the complete lecture word for word is not recommended because there is the danger of reading the lecture to the audience. It is better to have an outline; it allows the freedom to expand or reduce the content if time becomes an issue. Again, having timing cues on the notes will help you to keep track of the time you have left. Using PowerPoint makes it easy to update lectures and to tailor the lecture to a specific audience (see Tables 5.1 and 5.2 for examples of detailed and outlined lecture notes). However, even with PowerPoint, there is the risk of merely reading the content on the slides. To avoid this, use bullet points on the slides covering the key points to guide your lecture.

Practice

Practicing the delivery of the lecture before you give it will make the content flow more easily and help time the presentation. Practice using unfamiliar equipment to avoid frustrations.

Delivery

Voice

Make sure to articulate clearly and to speak loudly. Use a microphone if necessary. Students cannot hear or will miss important information if they are straining to listen. Refusing to use a microphone will be self-defeating.

TABLE 5.1   Detailed Lecture Notes

Testing for Creativity: Although many studies have been done to demonstrate that creativity and intelligence are not correlated, some researchers doubt some of the results on the basis of their belief that what is being measured is actually intelligence rather than creativity. For example, some critics say that the "Remote Associations" test is a test of convergent thinking rather than divergent thinking. (Ask what the group thinks is the difference between intelligence and creativity.)

TABLE 5.2   Outlined Lecture Notes

Future research directions:

- Methods of fostering creativity
- Discriminating between intelligence and creativity
- Larger samples
- Replication (remember to give a plug for this in general as a research activity)
- Longitudinal studies

If you think that using a microphone from a podium feels restrictive, find out ahead of time if the microphone can be hand-held or clipped to your lapel or collar. Be sure to clip the microphone to the side you will be facing the most; this will keep the sound and volume of your voice even. Always remember to turn off the microphone when your lecture is completed. (Many public speakers have told stories about forgetting to turn off the microphone while visiting the restroom or having a private conversation that was projected to an audience accidently.)

Humor

Do not tell jokes during lectures, but use examples of situations that are humorous.

Language

We have a tendency to use many abbreviations or acronyms when we interact and communicate within our health care setting. Be careful to avoid overuse of abbreviations in your lectures, and ensure that your students are aware of the terms you are using. If multiple abbreviations are needed to present the information effectively, consider giving the students a handout with a legend to refer to as you are speaking. Avoid the use of slang, and be careful not to use offensive language, even in jest.

Pace

Talk at a pace that will allow the students to both listen and take notes. Keep up the pace needed to cover the material without overloading the listeners. Some students may begin asking questions, indicating that they have an individual problem with the material, or the questions may pertain to material outside the purpose of the lecture. If it is obvious that many students have the same questions, answer them and try to make up lost time in some other way. However, if the questions seem important to only one or two students, talk with them after class.

Closing

It helps to emphasize the most significant point of the lecture by closing with an example illustrating important concepts. Summarize and hit the high points of the lecture.

Body Language

Body language is something to consider when lecturing. Smile and let students know that the content is interesting and important. Maintain eye contact with the entire class and not just students in the first row. In the beginning, this takes conscious effort, but it becomes easier over time. Gestures, such as touching one's hair or face, can be very distracting. Students have been known to count the number of times they observe specific behaviors rather than pay attention.

Appearance

Faculty members feel more confident about delivering a lecture when they are secure about their personal appearance. Select clothing that is comfortable, flattering, and professional. Make sure makeup is applied in a flattering way. Check your appearance before starting to ensure that is does not distract the learner or detract from the information you are presenting. To avoid visual overstimulation in your appearance, be conscious of wardrobe choices. If you are wearing clothing that has a bold pattern, then avoid adding bold jewelry or accessories.

If you are lecturing in a large room to a large group, make certain that the background contrasts with the color of your clothing. If the backdrop is lightly colored, wear something colorful. If the backdrop is brown or beige, choose something lighter or darker to provide contrast. Because of the potential risk of spreading germs, do not wear a uniform or laboratory coat that was worn in the clinical area. Change clothes before coming to school.

If you will be recorded on camera (for film or for Web presentations), avoid wearing white or light colors. Solid blue, red, or darker colors are recommended.

Media

It is beyond the scope of this book to go into much detail about media software and hardware; however, a few suggestions follow.

Hardware

Review the operation of the hardware prior to using it. Keep in mind that using the equipment goes with the territory of teaching and is just as important as knowing how to use the equipment and skills that go along with any kind of clinical nursing. Prior to giving the lecture, make sure the equipment used in your presentation is working. Keep the number of the audio-visual contact person with you, just in case you need help. Keep extra batteries on hand for microphones, laser pointers, and remote controls. A technical malfunction during the presentation will distract the listeners and cause you to loose momentum. Being prepared will keep you on track. (See Chapter 12 for more on the use of technology.)

Commercially Prepared Media

If you have rented or purchased commercially prepared media, know the media before using it. Give the students an adequate introduction before showing a film or videotaped presentation so they will know what they should be getting out of viewing the material. Afterward, emphasize the important points and discuss how they relate to the content.

Handouts

Printed material should look polished and professional. If a handout has the faculty name and the name of the school on it, it should look as neat and thoughtfully constructed as possible. When putting together a handout, keep in mind that students may keep it for a long time if it contains useful information.

Make sure the handout clearly conveys what is intended. Sometimes students receive handouts that contradict their readings or the lectures.

If there are discrepancies that need to be cleared up with these additional data, make sure the students know which reference to use. If the handout is related to some type of process, make sure the process is clearly explained.

If the handouts are made from a PowerPoint presentation, you may consider how many slides per page are appropriate. If the faculty member is posting the handout online for the students to print, and are posting it in a pdf version, the student will not be able to change the number of slides per printed page. For example, if the presentation is 100-slides long, and the handout has 3 slides per page, the student will be required to print 33 pages. Alternatively, the faculty member may choose to post the content outline view from the PowerPoint slides.

Producing Media

When using slides, computer programs, or overhead projections to convey information, take time in producing media, or ask for assistance from a technician to prepare the media effectively. Using a slide, PowerPoint projection, or transparency that is too busy is almost worse than using nothing at all. Students struggle to decipher cryptic handwriting or to find the minute structure in the illustration.

One of the most basic rules about projected media is to keep it simple. Yet, time after time, copies are made from a standard 8-1/2 x 11-inch piece of paper, and students sitting 10 or more rows away are expected to be able to distinguish line 7 from line 17.

On projected media, limit text to six or seven lines. A rule of thumb is 7 x 7—seven words per line, seven lines per slide. Use large print, or use a copy machine that can increase the size of the original. Use single words or short phrases rather than long sentences or paragraphs.

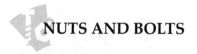

NUTS AND BOLTS

Expert Lecturers

Attend lectures by people who students say are good lecturers. Watch what they do and how they do it. Talk to colleagues about how they prepare and specifically how they deal with aspects of the process that are difficult.

Speech and Drama Experts

People with expertise in other fields can share things that are useful in lecturing. For example, speech teachers and drama coaches can help formally and informally in identifying techniques that will increase effectiveness as a lecturer. These colleagues can help with voice projection or timing to convey a particular emphasis.

Coteaching

To avoid getting into competition with a colleague or ending up suffering by comparison, work closely with that person in preparation and planning for the actual delivery of the lecture. One person may deliver some of the factual information while the other provides clinical illustrations or vice versa. Make a contract with each other to give and receive input about lecture style.

Evaluating Yourself

Make arrangements to have a lecture videotaped and ask a colleague to review it. This technique is helpful in evaluating verbal delivery by listening to pace, use of language, timing, and so forth.

Be certain to analyze body movements, eye contact, and other aspects of style that may contribute to or detract from effectiveness.

If you have lectured on a topic for a long time, you may be stuck in a rut. In your self-evaluation, consider if you are using the most appropriate material and the best presentation style. Revising your information, reevaluating current literature, and updating the type of media used will freshen the presentation, not only for the students, but for you, too.

FINAL WORDS

Giving lectures is the most common teaching method. As with many things we all do, we tend to take it for granted and do not consider how much is involved in the process. No matter how good we are, we can probably improve our style by being aware. Remember that the student audience has paid for an education. As a role model for the profession, present knowledge with skill and style.

FURTHER READING

Bligh, D. (2000). *What is the use of lectures?* San Francisco: Jossey-Bass.

Moravec, M., Williams, A., Aguilar-Roca, N., & O'Dowd, D. K. (2010). Learn before lecture: A strategy that improves learning outcomes in a large introductory biology class. *CBE-Life Sciences Education, 9*(4), 473–481. doi:10.1187/cbe.10–04–0063

6

Planning a Successful Seminar

A seminar is a group discussion with the objective of promoting learning among the participants. It enables students to learn to synthesize and use complex information. A successful seminar is a planned discussion for the dissemination of information that allows students to practice critical thinking skills. Research has demonstrated that people learn more effectively when they have an active role in the process of learning. A seminar has a small group of students, and everyone is asked to actively participate.

Learning should be an active process. Introducing the seminar learning method in the classroom complements more traditional teaching strategies such as didactic lecture and makes learning more interesting. A seminar gives the student the opportunity to take information from lectures, reading, clinical practice, and other experiences and to use that information to solve problems. The exchange of ideas becomes an active process among students and increases the students' knowledge of the topic. In today's world, students want learning to be exciting and engaging. The most crucial thing directly related to the thrill of learning seems to be the desire to learn. Faculty members need to find ways to increase students' desire to learn as much as to provide the students with the information they need. A seminar is a method that enables faculty to stimulate their desire to learn and to get them directly involved in the teaching and learning process.

A seminar usually last 1 to 3 hours and can take on a variety of forms. Students in the classroom may be divided into groups to work on case studies, which can then be presented to the entire class. Readings are assigned, content may be presented, and then students work in groups. Knowledge is applied using a case-study approach and then shared with the class. Another approach is where the course content is presented to a large class of students in a lecture format. Then the class is divided into small groups (8–10 students) for small-group seminars related to the content that has been presented along with course readings. Depending on the class size, the appropriate number of faculty is assigned for the seminars. This approach is faculty intensive and may not be feasible in all institutions. The advantage of this approach is that each faculty member presents lecture content related to his or her area of expertise during the semester and is also involved in the weekly seminars. This approach works well for content related to evidence-based practice, research, ethics, and communication.

An afternoon of clinical time may be used to provide an opportunity for students to learn through seminar. This is a good time to bring in practicing nurses, advanced practice nurses, respiratory therapists, physical therapists, and professionals from other disciplines that students may collaborate with during their clinical day. Keep in mind that professionals from other disciplines may not have recent experience with seminar-type learning, so objectives and the process must be clear to all. For example, a dietician may present information to students who will then break into groups for discussion. At the end, students may present a summary of their discussion to their peers and to their instructor. The dietician may participate by posing questions and making comments to the groups.

ONLINE SEMINARS

Most electronic learning platforms can support some type of simulated seminar activity. Blackboard uses discussion boards; Moodle uses forums. Both can be used for a modified version of a seminar, and the discussion will be asynchronous. With this type of discussion, the faculty member can post the seminar topic and set the ground rules. These rules may include the number of times one has to respond to postings, the length of time the discussion will be conducted, and the grading criteria, if any. Depending on the size of class, you may decide to use the general discussion board and allow all students to participate in the same seminar group. If the class size is large, then another option is to divide the class into groups and use the group discussion boards. Each group will have their own discussion board, and it will not be visible to the other groups. The advantage of the group discussion board for a seminar activity is that the group is small, and so it allows for better interaction among the students to contribute new ideas. With the general discussion board and a large class, most ideas may have been presented before all students have had an opportunity to contribute to the discussion. An additional strategy is to ask each student to post a comment or response to the seminar topic or question before a predetermined time and date. Then, after this time but before a designated end date, the student has to respond to perhaps two colleagues' postings. This assists the discussion and keeps the students engaged in the seminar. For a synchronous experience, live chat can be used. One advantage of the online format is that students who would ordinarily hesitate to speak in front of a group may feel more comfortable online. Students must be given clear instruction in the use of the technology and be familiar with the ways to participate in the discussion (i.e., to raise their electronic hand). An electronic format may be better suited for upper division or graduate students but can also be introduced to lower division students. Most critical for the online version of a seminar is that the teacher be proficient with the technology and be able to give detailed instructions and expectations to the learners.

GOALS

Seminars are used to increase student involvement in the learning process. The seminar approach is useful in helping students attain high-level cognitive objectives, such as analysis, synthesis, and evaluation. This approach also promotes the achievement of affective objectives.

TOOLS

Objectives

At the beginning of the seminar learning experience it is important to set the objectives the students should accomplish. Keep the level of the students in mind in order to write appropriate objectives. A seminar is most appropriate in courses that have high-level cognitive objectives. Seminars, although not generally used in lower division courses, may be useful if there is a structured approach. Develop some key questions to guide the seminar in order to facilitate learning for lower division classes that might have little experience using seminars. Limit objectives to about four or five for a 2-hour seminar.

Objectives should provide the foundation for the outcomes of the seminar. Objectives relating only to knowledge and comprehension are usually inappropriate for seminars, because they only require the students to regurgitate information rather than to analyze and discuss the information. Verbs such as *analyze, evaluate, explain, formulate, generalize, integrate, organize, solve,* and *synthesize* would be appropriate.

Content

The activities to be covered in the seminar should be provided to the students in a hardcopy or electronic handout. The seminar may include a presentation from the faculty member followed by discussion. This provides an opportunity for discussion of new content in a seminar. Be specific about the activities students should accomplish. Clear guidelines are essential for a successful seminar with achievement of seminar objectives. Table 6.1 shows a sample seminar guide.

Some seminar activities are used (1) to provide a series of critical discussion questions related to the objectives; (2) to make a list of points drawn from the objectives for the students to discuss; or (3) to include an exercise, a simulation, a presentation of new material, or other guided experience to stimulate discussion.

Process

Getting Started

The first step in the seminar process is that the faculty member is responsible for preparing and supporting students throughout the seminar. This begins with setting up ground rules for behavior. An effective way to do this is to have agreed-upon rules with the students.

The discussion about ground rules should include the seminar start and end time, student preparation and participation, and forms of presentation. It is useful to establish individual roles within a group (such as timekeeper) and perhaps dividing individual work assignments. Ground rules should also look at valuing other students' opinions and maintaining confidentiality. Each student is expected to participate

TABLE 6.1 Seminar Guide

Dealing With Special Group Problems

Objectives:

1. Develop an awareness of the individual and group needs that lead to special group problems.
2. Analyze the effects of selected problems.
3. Identify ways of intervening to deal with group problems.
4. Evaluate the outcomes of interventions used to deal with group problems.

Reading Assignment:

Faculty member inserts the selected assignment.

Students may refer to notes or handouts on specific content related to the seminar topic presented at the beginning of the seminar.

Process:

Consider the following special group problems in your discussion: monopolizing, scapegoating, silence, new members, absences, and manipulation.

1. Discuss each problem in the list using the seminar objectives.
2. How do you feel when you are in a group where these problems exist?
3. How would you feel about being the group leader and dealing with these problems?
4. With which problems would you feel the most and the least confident in intervening?

---

in the seminar. These rules will provide structure and safety for the group discussion. See Table 6.2 for a list of possible ground rules. If the group will meet for several seminars, it is useful to specify ground rules for the meetings. A copy of these rules should be given to each participant.

Stimulating Discussion

Faculty can assist in stimulating discussion by leading with an open-ended question or a declarative statement. Some seminar formats will involve a faculty presentation of content at the beginning of the class time followed by a seminar related to that content. Careful planning for a seminar is essential to manage and facilitate a discussion on a specific topic. Clearly, the seminar topic and opening discussion should be

TABLE 6.2   Seminar Ground Rules

1. The seminar will start on time, and everyone is expected to be present at the start of the seminar.
2. Each student must participate actively in the discussion.
3. Discussion will conclude at least 15 minutes before the end of the assigned seminar time in order to permit a summary.
4. Each student will have a turn to summarize the discussion.

relevant to the group at large. Broad topics, such as communication, group dynamics, evidence-based practice topics, and ethical issues are ideal seminar topics because they span clinical specialties, enabling students with different clinical experiences to relate the seminar topic to their experiences.

While ground rules provide a foundation for student participation, advice and cueing are two strategies that may enhance student participation, reinforce behavior, and provide feedback. With students who may be new to discussion activities, consider modeling for them the types of information that is appropriate and valuable for sharing.

Ask open-ended questions rather than questions easily answered with one- or two-word responses. For example, it would be more productive to ask, "What was the most uncomfortable experience you ever had with one of these problems?" rather than to ask, "Which of these problems makes you the most uncomfortable?"

When students participate and share ideas, reinforce this behavior by commenting on it. For example, "That is a good idea," "That has got us off to a good start," or "What do the rest of you think about Emma's point? Let's hear about your experiences with this issue."

Encouraging Appropriate Participation

Two of the most common participation problems are the students who talk too much and the students who talk too little. At the outset, set expectations about participation. One strategy is to specify the number of times each student is expected to make a substantive contribution to the discussion. However, you must be clear that quantity does not substitute for quality. Individual differences should be acknowledged. Some people are more talkative and more comfortable about talking than are others, but both kinds of people can learn from monitoring their own and others' behaviors.

Specify that students who are more comfortable at talking can help by giving the quieter students time to talk, and quieter students can take advantage of this opportunity to practice in a nonthreatening situation. It will help to remind the whole group that these are the stated expectations without necessarily putting particular people on the spot. Emphasize that everyone in the group is responsible for the group's outcome.

Limit the students from bringing outside people, such as guest faculty, to the group. Outsiders change the process of a group and may interfere with the regular group members' abilities to participate appropriately. Even though guest speakers who are experts on the topic may appear to be a good resource, it is usually more appropriate for the students to interview these people and share their findings rather than to invite them to the group. Media should be used with discretion; it should be used to effectively stimulate discussion rather than merely to consume group time. A short video or audio clip may be appropriate. Again, providing clear guidelines before the seminar regarding the use of media is important.

Staying on the Topic

Another gate-keeping function is helping the group to stay on the topic. Do not get too distressed if the group goes off on a tangent. Sometimes the tangents may be more productive than what was planned. However, if the group strays from objectives and seems to be slow about getting back to the point, say something like, "Okay, let's get back to the objectives," or "Let's get back on track." Do it with a normal tone of voice and a smile that conveys interest in the group's learning and not upset or frustrated that they have strayed from the topic.

If the group develops a tendency to stray from the topic every time they are together, assess what they keep talking about when they ignore the seminar topics. For example, if the group also is in a clinical course together, they may continually bring up things from clinical that do not relate to the seminar goals. This may be because they do not have adequate time to deal with the impact of clinical experiences. One possible solution would be to allot some time at the beginning of each seminar to clear the air about what is on their minds. Another solution could be to find time for them to deal with such concerns outside of the seminar. Also, at the beginning of each seminar, quickly revisit the seminar ground rules and the importance of staying on topic in relation to the objectives.

Correcting Misinformation

When students read about a particular topic for the first time, they may get an incorrect notion about what they have read. Other students may misread things or recall situations that were not accurate examples of what they were discussing. It is important to correct these erroneous ideas without seeming to put the student down for misunderstanding. If the misinformation is a common way for people to get mixed up, emphasize this so the group can avoid the same sort of problem in the future. A key faculty role in the seminar is active listening so that these types of misconceptions can be corrected in a supportive way before they become engrained in the students' minds.

Faculty might say the following: "Whoops. I think you got the variables reversed. A lot of people get independent and dependent variables mixed up. I think one reason is that in an experiment, you may be controlling the independent variable. It is hard to think of something that is being controlled as being independent. However, outside the experiment, that variable is not being controlled, and we think it affects the dependent variable in some way."

A straightforward explanation conveys important information and keeps the students' energy focused on meeting the objectives rather than on trying to regurgitate definitions. In a situation such as the one described, follow up with some examples and help the group to identify which variable is which in order to increase their confidence in dealing with the material. This emphasizes the importance of having expert faculty lead the seminar. They have the knowledge needed to present numerous examples to help students understand the material.

Sometimes a student has a vested interest in the piece of misinformation. The student may become caught up in trying to defend the information for personal reasons. Here your role is to redirect the students and to gently but firmly guide them toward correct information and ensure that they understand it.

Although it is likely that most instructors have distressed students inappropriately, it sometimes may actually promote learning to encourage students to be distressed about not knowing the correct answer. For example, if there is controversy about the right answer, ask the students to look further for the correct answers and bring them back to the seminar. Additional resources such as journal articles and electronic sources may be provided to aid this process.

Drawing to Closure

Closure is another ground rule to establish. It helps to have a summary including the key points in the discussion or significant realizations the group has reached. For the first seminar, give the students an outline of what should be included in the summary. The summary helps to solidify the understandings gained from the discussion. It can also provide a direction for further discussions of the same topic or subsequent topics. For the first few seminars, provide constructive feedback on the quality of the summary so that the students become proficient in developing a seminar summary.

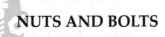

NUTS AND BOLTS

Leadership

Faculty members take on leadership responsibilities in a seminar with inexperienced students. Leadership in a seminar takes the form of facilitating the students through the process described earlier in this chapter. Advanced students can be expected to take on some of the leadership responsibilities, but the faculty member is ultimately responsible for helping to make this a positive learning experience.

If the students will be responsible for the facilitation, give them some guidance to get started. For example, assign a reading about the seminar process, or review the process as it is described in this chapter.

When students have leadership responsibilities, decide who will be responsible for each seminar. Planning this at the beginning of the semester gives students the opportunity to schedule ample time for preparation. Generally, two students work together. They can share the work for preparation as well as the tasks of facilitating the group. More than two students are inappropriate, because it is unrealistic to expect a group to function with the leadership responsibilities spread so thin.

Faculty members occasionally have unrealistic expectations of the sophistication of students in leadership roles. They may expect students to confront and deal with complex problems of participation without any faculty assistance. When there are problems either within one meeting or within the group as a whole, the faculty member needs to step in and help to bring the problems into the open for discussion. The faculty member needs to be vigilant to identify problems or issues early and nip them in the bud, otherwise the seminar learning process will fail due to lack of guidance and attention to the ground rules.

Evaluation

In some situations, it may be appropriate to evaluate and grade seminars. Evaluation may be based on the students' meeting the objectives adequately in relation to content, as well as evaluation of the process itself. The evaluation may be as basic as acknowledging that each objective was met and how. Develop an evaluation tool that integrates the content and the process. An example is given in Table 6.3.

For courses in which seminars constitute a major portion of the course activity, attach a grade to the evaluation. Generally, this is done when the course has important objectives that are met only through the seminar. A seminar grade is also more common when there is a significant weight placed on group process as a part of the framework of the curriculum.

If evaluating and grading the seminars in the course, be sure to keep the course objectives and their relative weights in mind. For example, if the seminars deal with major content and group process is significant, both content and process should be given significant weight in determining the students' course grades. In other situations, less may be expected of the students and less weight given to any evaluation and grade.

With students who are less experienced in seminar activities, the faculty member may start by doing the total evaluation. As the students gain more experience, they can begin to participate in the evaluation and eventually in the grading. Also, students may be encouraged to grade their individual performance following each seminar. This may take the form of a letter grade or, more constructively, the letter grade may be accompanied with a couple of sentences justifying their choice of letter grade. This grade may be submitted to the faculty member at the end of the seminar for faculty feedback on the student's individual performance.

Expect more from the outset from students who are experienced in seminars and grade them accordingly. With inexperienced seminar

TABLE 6.3   Seminar Evaluation Guide

Content:

1. Seminar objectives were met

    - 100% of objectives met
    - 90% of objectives met
    - 80% of objectives met
    - 70% of objectives met
    - Less than 70% of objectives met

2. Correct information was shared

    - 100% of information was complete and accurate
    - 90% of information was complete and accurate
    - 80% of information was complete and accurate
    - 70% of information was complete and accurate
    - Less than 70% of information was complete and accurate

3. Appropriate references were used

    - Assigned reading plus other resources
    - Assigned reading plus one other resource
    - Assigned reading only

4. Useful examples and experiences were shared

    - Many examples and experiences/anecdotes
    - Some examples and experiences/anecdotes
    - Few examples and experiences/anecdotes
    - No examples or experiences/anecdotes

Process:

1. The seminar started on time
2. All members participated
3. Participation was appropriate (i.e., no silent members, no monopolizing)
4. The group stayed on the assigned topic
5. If problems were present, the group dealt with them
6. A summary was presented
7. The seminar ended on time

participants or with a new group, grade more leniently in the first few meetings. Try to be realistic about what your students can handle, given their backgrounds. Remember, the seminar is a learning strategy and it is important to encourage the students with constructive criticism along with the letter grade. As the students gain experience in the seminar format, the grading criteria may be made more stringent.

When students participate in the grading, allot different percentages to how much the faculty member and the students contribute to the final grade. Separate the process grade from the content grade. For example, in one situation, the students and faculty each contributed one third of the grade based on the achievement of content. The last third was contributed only by faculty and was based on the faculty member's evaluation of the group's ability to evaluate their own process. The formula is presented in Table 6.4.

If the formula outlined in Table 6.4 is used, the main control of the grade is left with the faculty, although the students can certainly influence the grade. Part of the students' evaluation could include some points on their own evaluation of their group process. This approach is especially appropriate in courses where group process and change are important aspects. Because the faculty member evaluates the students on their abilities to recognize and try to correct their problems, they can partially improve their grade if they are honest and insightful in their self-evaluation. Alternatively, the self-evaluation is not part of the official seminar grade but is used to help the student's self-development. You can decide whether you wish to include the student's individual grade in the total grade. Guiding principles may be the importance of getting honest, useful self-assessments that can be used to enhance the learning, and whether the individual grade is a critical part of the total seminar process.

Trying to grade individuals in a seminar is complex. Although it seems a good idea to evaluate each individual separately, it is difficult to do fairly. To give some credit for individual preparation for the seminar, require a bibliography on the assigned reading or give a short quiz related to the reading assignment. Remember that the written word requires more time to read, comment, and grade. Another strategy that may be more appealing is to set aside time in the seminar for

TABLE 6.4　Group-Grade Calculation Formula

Content: A = faculty grade; B = student grade

Evaluation process: C = faculty grade

Seminar grade = (A + B + C) divided by 3

Example: (93% + 95% + 98%) divided by 3 = 95.33%

the students to share their bibliographies, or have the students grade each other's quizzes and use the information when they proceed with their discussion.

FINAL WORDS

Seminars can be effective ways to facilitate achievement of high-level objectives. Careful planning and facilitation leads to a successful seminar. Seminar participation assists in developing critical thinking skills and understanding of the dynamics of group process. This method of teaching allows for an active and shared responsibility toward creating a goal-oriented learning experience.

FURTHER READING

Rowles, C. J., & Russo, B. L. (2009). Strategies to promote critical thinking and active learning. In D. M. Billings & J. A. Halstead (Eds.), *Teaching in nursing: A guide for faculty* (3rd ed., pp. 238–261). St. Louis, MO: Elsevier.

Stiles, A. S., Johnson, R. K., Trigg, B. K., & Fowler, G. (2004). Cooperative learning: The ugly, the bad, and the good. *Nurse Educator, 29,* 97–98.

Xakellis, G. C., Richner, S., & Stevenson, F. (2005). Comparison of knowledge acquired by students in small group seminars with and without a formal didactic component. *Medical Student Education, 37,* 27–29.

7

Course Design, Implementation, and Evaluation

The more time and effort invested into designing a course, the fewer problems when it is implemented. Even a fairly standard course, such as a medical-surgical nursing course, will need work toward putting it together in a logical and useful way.

The first time a faculty member is asked to teach, he or she is usually not expected to design the course. However, the new faculty member will soon need to know how to do this. Rather than copying another faculty member's design for another course in the curriculum, know the principles involved. Faculty groups that are interested in designing a new course often will work together rather than have a single faculty member work alone. However, if a faculty member does work alone, he or she should ask for input and feedback from colleagues.

It is easier to describe the course design process in the order that will eventually show up in a course syllabus. Start by listing the content that should go into the course and then write the course description. The curriculum committee must approve course descriptions and course objectives, so do not make changes unless you have approval. Make sure that you are working with the latest version approved by the curriculum committee.

GOALS

Effective course design facilitates the presentation of content. Attention to design makes it possible to acquaint students from the outset with the direction and expectations of the course.

TOOLS

Curriculum Context

Theoretical Model

Whether or not the curriculum is based on a well-known model, there is a framework around which it is organized. Most schools have a content map. The elements of the model, content map, and framework dictate the organization of each of the courses. Before trying to design the course, understand the context.

In many nursing curricula, the major organizing concepts are person (or humanity), environment, health (or health and illness), and nursing. To some extent, each course in the curriculum reflects these concepts, advances the students' understanding of them individually, and promotes the students' grasp of the interrelationships.

Usually, the organizing concepts are defined in the school's philosophy. Although there are diverse definitions, there are also similarities in which aspects of these concepts are described. *Person* is described as an individual, perhaps in terms of interactions with others. The person may be described as an independent, dependent, or interdependent organism. If the school is part of a sectarian college, the relationship of the person to a higher power may be included.

Environment describes the milieu in which the person and nursing intersect. *Health* or *health and illness* will be described in terms of the impact of nursing intervention. *Nursing* is described in relation to the scope of practice and its place as a profession.

Placement

The year in which the students are expected to take the course determines the complexity of the course design. Courses early in the curriculum will be based on simpler objectives. Generally, courses should move from the simple to the complex and from the normal to the abnormal. Establish where the students are in their program, and review their level of knowledge. Check the curriculum, and identify previous course content that will impact the course. This information will help when making decisions related to the type and amount of content that is required in the course. If the content has been presented in a previous course, then a quick review may be all that is needed.

Prerequisites

The course must be placed so that students will have completed appropriate prerequisites in order to be able to understand the new content. For example if the requirement is for the students to know complex pharmacology, but complex pharmacology is not taught in the course, place it after they have taken the appropriate pharmacology courses. By the same token, do not repeat content or assignments already tackled in a prerequisite course unless there is a new application that students need to learn.

If the course is meant to be prerequisite to other courses, make sure to include the content students will need when they get to those other courses. For example, if the course is supposed to prepare students to develop teaching care plans, and other courses do not offer this information, include that content and the application of teaching and learning principles in the prerequisite course.

Strands

Another common feature of nursing curricula is strands, or threads, that are woven throughout and help to support major concepts. These strands often include the following: nutrition, pharmacology, professionalism, individual/family/group, acute/rehabilitative/chronic care, hospital/community settings, and primary/secondary/tertiary prevention. These strands vary according to the other organizing elements in the framework, but whatever they are within the curriculum, consider how to incorporate them into the course. Not every course will include all of the strands. For example, nutrition and pharmacology might not be found in a course on nursing trends and issues. However, the strand of professionalism would be the predominant theme in that course. When designing the course, review the curriculum to see the content of the strands and the existing courses that incorporate this content. The faculty member will decide which strands are relevant for the new course and consciously include the strand content in the course.

Course Delivery Formats

When designing a course, consider the method of course delivery. Will the teaching and learning take place in the classroom, online, in the clinical setting, in the laboratory, or in some combinations of these formats? The type of delivery will alter aspects of the design such as the teaching strategies, evaluation, and perhaps interaction with the students. Currently, many courses are offered online or are hybrid in nature, with some content offered face to face and other content offered online. With mixed-delivery formats, the faculty member can engage students with most of the usual teaching strategies such as lecture, asynchronous and synchronous discussion, group work, and student presentations and projects.

Syllabus Format

Usually a course will have an established format to follow. Look at the way other courses are set up, especially how the syllabi for similar courses are organized. This will establish the pattern for designing the course.

An abbreviated sample of a syllabus format is shown in Table 7.1. In addition to the introductory information furnished in the sample, attach guides for the course's required assignments and evaluation.

TABLE 7.1   Format for a Course Syllabus

Beta University, Alpha School of Nursing

N321 Psychiatric Mental Health Nursing

Course Description: Focus is on the use of the nursing process with acutely ill psychiatric patients in an inpatient setting. Emphasis is on the use of self in promoting therapeutic nurse/patient relationships. Experience is limited to working with adults.

Placement in Curriculum: Junior standing; prerequisites N232 and N237

(continued)

TABLE 7.1 *(continued)*

Conceptual Framework: Psychiatric/mental health nurses use interpersonal communication skills and the nursing process to assist persons who are temporarily dependent due to severe psychiatric/emotional problems interfering with their mental health. Strands addressed in this course include research, pharmacology, professionalism, individual/family/group, acute/rehabilitative/chronic care, hospital/community settings, and primary/secondary/tertiary prevention.

Course Objectives: At the end of this course, the student will be able to complete the following:

1. Describe the use of the nursing process with psychiatric patients.
2. Identify and implement therapeutic nursing interventions for use with adult psychiatric patients.
3. Differentiate between nursing practice with psychiatric patients and the practice of other mental health workers.

Required Text: Keltner, N., Schweche, L. & Bostrom, C. (2003). *Psychiatric nursing* (5th ed.). St. Louis, MO: Mosby. (ISBN 0–323–03906–5)

Evaluation and Grading: The theory grade will be determined by the student's performance on two tests and a comprehensive final examination. The student's clinical performance and the written nursing case study will determine the clinical grade. Students will be formally evaluated at midterm and at the end of the term using the evaluation tool included in the syllabus.

Theory: Test 1 = 15%

Test 2 = 15%

Final = 20%

Clinical: Performance = 35%

Case study = 15%

Students must receive a passing grade in both clinical and theory before the grades are averaged for the course grade. A failure in either part of the course constitutes a failure in the course.

Content:	*Assigned Reading:*
Conceptual Framework	Chapters 1–3
Therapeutic Use of Self	Chapters 4, 10, 13
Nursing Process	Chapters 11–12
Patterns of Anxiety	Chapters 29–31
Depression and Elation	Chapters 34–36

Consistent patterns in course format help in preparing self-study reports for state approval as well as for Commission on Collegiate Nursing Education (CCNE) or National League for Nursing Accrediting Commission (NLNAC) reports.

Course Description

The course description gives a concise overview, describes the principal focus, and identifies the major teaching methodologies. An example would be as follows:

Nursing Concepts 1. Introduction to the systematic use of the nursing process in selected clinical settings. Focus is on the individual, with major emphasis on alterations in fluid/electrolyte balance, acid/base status, and blood composition. Needs in the following areas are addressed: comfort/sleep, oxygenation, nutrition, elimination, mobility, grieving, aging, and dying. Practical laboratory experience includes acquisition of health assessment techniques and clinical experience in hospital and extended-care facilities.

This course description would be appropriate for course materials, but some colleges and universities require shorter descriptions for the catalog. If it is necessary to shorten the description, try to make it convey as much as possible in the words allowed. The original is 68 words long. It would be possible to write a shorter version, with only 39 words, without losing anything significant:

Nursing Concepts 1. Introduction to the systematic use of the nursing process with individuals experiencing alterations in fluid/electrolytes, acid/base, blood, and human functioning needs. Practical experience includes acquisition of health assessment techniques and clinical experience in hospital and extended-care facilities.

Neither of these descriptions constitutes timeless prose, but they do a fair job of telling a prospective student or anyone else something about the course. Even a novice or outsider could probably grasp the meaning of the words used in this context.

Course Objectives

The objectives proceed logically from the course description and should be written with consideration for the elements listed under the section Curriculum Context. Because the course description in the example is obviously for a beginning-level course, consider writing objectives on the lower cognitive levels pertaining to knowledge, comprehension, and application. Some examples are shown in Table 7.2. The objectives in the table are written in behavioral terms that are measurable. Review the course objectives carefully, and revise and develop new ones if needed. The curriculum committee usually has to pass changes to these objectives. More specific objectives can be created from these course objectives for each class or clinical experience (see Table 7.2). The faculty member develops the class objectives and can change them each time the course is taught.

Content

Organize the content in the order reflected by the objectives or in the chronological order in which it will be covered. Make sure the content is on the appropriate level, and match the content level to the level of the student. As in the example in Table 7.2, if blood disorders need to be addressed, limit the depth for a beginning-level course. On the

TABLE 7.2   Course Objectives

At the conclusion of this course, the student will be able to complete the following:

1. Describe each step in the nursing process
2. Demonstrate beginning ability to use the nursing process in working with individual clients
3. Apply the nursing process in working with individuals with alterations in fluid/electrolyte balance, acid/base status, and blood composition
4. Use the nursing process in addressing needs in the areas of human functioning, such as comfort/sleep, oxygenation, nutrition, elimination, and mobility
5. Identify and respond to nursing care needs for individuals who are grieving, aging, and dying
6. Demonstrate competent and safe use of health assessment techniques

other hand, the students will be unengaged if the content is presented at too low a level for them.

Reading Assignments

The following chapter deals with the selection of texts and making reading assignments, but these tasks also need to be considered while planning the course. If a textbook has been chosen, consider organizing the course content in the same order as in the book. This will make it easier for the students to use.

Evaluation and Grading of Students

Decide how to evaluate the students' achievement of the course objectives. Relate these methods to the level of the course objectives. The course should constitute a reasonable amount of work for the credits assigned to the course. A combination of major and minor assignments and examinations is advised. The details of selecting and using these tools are described in later chapters, but include the relevant information for the students in the course syllabus. The information should include the number and type of assignments, the due dates, and the percentage course grade for each assignment.

Teaching Methodology

Determine the most effective teaching strategies that will maximize student learning. Plan to use a wide range of teaching strategies that will engage students and meet their different learning styles. Match the teaching strategies to the course objectives and the curriculum objectives. The lecture method is most efficient with objectives that are mostly in the cognitive realm and on the levels of knowledge, comprehension, and application. However, the lecture used alone is a passive learning strategy. The faculty member should strive to include some active learning strategies such as discussion to stimulate student thinking. If dealing with higher cognitive levels of analysis, synthesis, and evaluation or if dealing with objectives in the affective domain, methods such as seminar will better enable the students to practice meeting such objectives. Psychomotor objectives can best be met by the students' having practice laboratory or clinical experiences. Clinical experiences in most nursing courses will provide an opportunity for addressing objectives at different levels in any domain, but the expectations will be simpler in the first courses as contrasted with the more advanced courses in the curriculum.

Course Evaluation

Course evaluation is the responsibility of the faculty, with input from the students. Plan for the evaluation of the course from the start and fit it into the system used by the school. If there are components of the course that need special evaluation, add them to the tool being used within the program. Be sure to allow class time for students to evaluate the course and the faculty who teach it.

Faculty members may like to receive feedback after each class. One option is to have students complete anonymously a 1-minute feedback sheet with three or four questions, such as "What was the 'muddiest point' today in class? What went well? What did you not like? Any other comments you would like to make?" This informal feedback is invaluable as the faculty member has the opportunity at the beginning of the next class to address any misunderstandings or any part of the content that appears unclear before moving ahead to new content. Also, the faculty can change anything in the class that is not working. Students like to give this type of feedback, particularly if the faculty member is responsive. Overall, this quick, 1-minute feedback at the end of class is a good gauge of how the class is going.

In addition to the students' evaluations, keep a log or file of faculty perceptions of the components of the course. For example, after giving a lecture, the decision that the content was too complex might be made. Write that down with ideas about how to change in the future. Use this evaluation of the course and the summary of the students' evaluations to determine what needs to be changed and how.

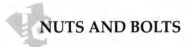

NUTS AND BOLTS

Guest Speakers or Experts

As a new faculty member, you may be the only resource for the majority of the responsibilities entailed in implementing the course. However, do not hesitate to enlist the help of other nursing faculty members for some classes as well as practicing nurses outside the faculty. For example, invite a nursing faculty member who specializes in ethics to lecture on ethical implications within the scope of the course.

There is a lot of work involved in developing lectures for 15 weeks of class. Although teaching from the area of expertise, it still takes time to put together cohesive lectures that will help the students meet the objectives. Get the help of a local expert to do a lecture if needed. For example, if you are teaching a course in psychiatric nursing, and the faculty member has little experience in the treatment of substance abuse, invite a clinical nursing specialist in the field to lecture on this topic.

Before asking a guest to lecture on a topic, ascertain that person's ability to speak in public. A lot of people are nervous about speaking to a group. Their anxiety may result in failing to address objectives. They might run over the allotted time or run too short, leaving the students in a bind either way. If possible, listen to the potential guest speaker ahead of time. If this cannot be arranged, find someone trusted to evaluate the prospective speaker.

Sometimes it will not be possible to validate speaking ability ahead of time, so be prepared for some predictable problems. The first way to avoid trouble is to contact the guest well in advance. Discuss what the guest will address and share the lecture objectives in writing. If this lecture is for an online class, explain the logistics to the guest speaker. There may be the option of taping the class in advance and having a synchronized discussion at the end of the session (see Chapter 12). Suggest another brief chat prior to the lecture so the guest speaker can tell you what he or she plans to talk about. Give the guest the ground rules in writing, such as the starting time for the class, when to give breaks, if appropriate, and when to end the class. Discuss how the guest will handle student questions, including when to get back to covering the planned material.

Find out in advance if the guest will require any media support. Once the parameters are agreed upon, send a letter that validates the plans. Include all the particulars, including equipment that will be available. Give explicit directions about the location and parking.

A week before the guest is expected, send an email or phone call to touch base and find out if there are any questions or problems. Validate that the guest will be able to find the classroom or know where to meet in order to go to the classroom together. It is a courteous to meet the guest a little before class time. Go to your office and share some refreshments or otherwise make the guest feel welcome and at home. Usually, faculty will not be in a position to offer the guest any remuneration for this service, so little personal gestures and attention to details can do a lot to show genuine gratitude for the expert speaker's contribution.

When introducing the guest to the students, share his or her credentials and why this person was chosen to lecture. Then turn the class over. Usually, things will go fine, even if the guest strays a bit or does not address every objective. Sometimes, if the class is large, discipline problems might occur. Remind students to be respectful and professional.

After the class, attend to details that show gratitude. Within a day or two, follow up with a note or letter thanking the guest. If possible, address something specific about the presentation to make the thank you personal. For example, "Your description of the teenage patient withdrawing from alcohol was especially powerful and instructive."

After the lecture, evaluate the guest to decide whether to make the same invitation in the future.

Organizing

No matter how helpful this or any other book may be in helping to prepare and present a course, seasoned colleagues on the faculty will be useful resources. Administrative or clerical staff is also invaluable in helping to figure out how things really work. Get to know the instructional technology and media staff; you will need their assistance, often at short notice when some of the technology fails. The responsibilities of a course coordinator may vary from school to school. The following responsibilities may be either faculty or those of other people. Figure out how the following are accomplished.

Requesting classrooms

Reserving instructional technology equipment

Securing instructional technology software

Arranging for clinical sites

Having your syllabus typed and duplicated

Selecting texts

Putting readings on reserve in the library

Arranging for journal articles to be available online and checking copyright rules

Arranging for guest speakers
Preparing your own lectures
Constructing tests and having them printed
Arranging for machine grading of tests
Grading assignments
Distributing midterm grade deficiencies
Counseling students with problems in the course
Reporting final grades
Arranging for course and faculty evaluation
Developing proficiency examinations

Institutional Policies

Be informed of institutional policies about the presentation of courses. These can usually be found in the catalog or a policy manual. Some of the issues affected by such policies follow. Check to see if there is an official policy before making a decision.

Beginning and ending dates of course
Class times (starting, stopping, and breaks)
Official holidays
Canceling or rescheduling classes
Numerical values of letter grades
Auditors in class
Dates for dropping or withdrawing from courses
Recipients of deficiency notices
Restrictions on and removal of incomplete grade
Recipients of official grade reports
Examination policies covering the following:
   Required exams
   Make-up exams
   Date of final exam
Credit by proficiency examination
Grievances

FINAL WORDS

Although designing a course may not be immediately required of new faculty, one can learn by watching how it has been done by other members. Eventually, this responsibility will be part of a new faculty-member's role. Although it is challenging at first, most faculty enjoy having this chance to be creative and to share their knowledge and expertise.

FURTHER READING

Billings, C. M., & Halstead, J. A. (2009). *Teaching in nursing: A guide for faculty* (3rd ed.). Philadelphia: Saunders.

Textbook and Reading Assignment Selection

N urse educators are charged with the responsibility of selecting textbooks and reading assignments that are congruent with tenets of professional nursing practice, national and global health priorities, cultural competencies, and the mission of their particular school of nursing. In addition, textbooks and reading assignments should link course content, empirical evidence, and application to practice. Given the large body of nursing literature available as traditional printed textbooks and the increasing amount available via Internet and digital technologies, the selection of textbooks and reading assignments can be a daunting task, even for the most experienced nursing faculty. In the 21st century, the knowledge base in all sciences and professions is expanding exponentially. There are approximately 1,500 journals reviewed and indexed in the *Cumulative Index of Nursing and Allied Health* alone. With new journals cropping up each year, it is difficult to keep up with the literature in your own field of nursing, let alone maintain a general currency of knowledge in all areas of nursing practice.

Many new editions of books include CD-ROMs or DVDs, test banks, laboratory manuals, online resources, and other helpful supplements. In any text, the author or editor must make choices about what can be included and in what depth the topics will be handled. An author also decides about the model or organizational framework used to present the content. These decisions must be considered when choosing textbooks for students. This chapter provides nursing faculty with a step-by-step approach for identifying, evaluating, selecting, and posting the best textbooks and journal reading assignments for their students.

GOALS

The principal goal for assigning textbook and reading material is to provide the students with accurate information on a given topic. In addition, reading assignments are commonly used to assist students in understanding the class material, to increase class participation, and to improve student test performance.

TOOLS

Textbook Selection and Evaluation

Textbook Sources

Although Internet sources and digital technologies increase at exponential rates, traditional textbooks continue to be an efficient way to present content areas in nursing. A study by the National Association of College Book Stores estimated that traditional textbooks continue to make up nearly 98% of all textbook sales. However, some analysts predict that by 2014, more than 20% of textbooks sales will be in e-book format.

Faculty should recognize that the majority of current undergraduate nursing students were born between 1980 and 2000, and they are considered millennial learners. Millennial learners have grown up with digital technologically and learn best with interactive technology. Although traditional textbooks and journal articles address course content effectively, faculty should increasingly look for reading assignments that are delivered with innovative and interactive technologies.

Evaluating Prospective Texts

Process Criteria

Before reviewing any texts, determine the criterion on which you will base your evaluation. Aside from evaluating the general content, consider all of the other factors that make a textbook valuable: Does the textbook follow a particular theorist's model? Does the textbook present global perspectives? Does the textbook foster cultural competence? In addition, the criterion should include evaluating the different methods the textbook uses to present information (e.g., illustrations, charts, algorithms, case-based studies, CDs, DVDs, test banks, laboratory manuals, etc.). Ideally, textbooks are expected to provide a framework for what is taught, how it is taught, and the sequence in which it is taught.

Table 8.1 includes a format that can be used to evaluate a text. The form may be used to evaluate a book in any clinical area of nursing. Rating the elements with a Likert scale from 0 (*unsatisfactory*) to (*excellent*) may be useful when comparing similar textbooks. Other items might be evaluated with a dichotomous scale of *yes* or *no.*

TABLE 8.1   Textbook Evaluation Form

Name of textbook_____

Publisher_____

Cost_____

Author_____

Publication date_____

Replaces text_____

General:

_____Conceptual framework harmonious with ours

_____Comprehensive

_____Emphasis on nursing models

_____Approach to nursing process consistent with ours

_____Definitions consistent with our terminology

_____Builds on prerequisite content

_____Aimed at students in upper division

_____Internally consistent

_____Nonsexist language

_____Useful index

(continued)

TABLE 8.1   Textbook Evaluation Form *(continued)*

Format:

_____Objectives given

_____Clear chapter introductions

_____Theory is current; recent reference citations

_____Nursing research is discussed and used

_____Clear examples are given to illustrate important points

_____Significant issues are emphasized

_____Headings enhance ease of finding material

_____Important content is highlighted

_____Photographs, tables, graphs, and diagrams

_____Summaries are succinct and recap important points

Readability:

_____Size and style of print promote ease of reading

_____Narrative style enhances reading

_____Appropriate reading level for course

_____Readability score

Instructional aids:

_____Instructor's manual available

_____Student workbook available

Media available:

    Specify types_____

Test-item bank available:

_____ Book format _____Computer software

Comments:

Content Criteria

Faculty should have a strong understanding of what they are looking for in a textbook. Aside from foundational knowledge, textbook content should be salient to nursing practice and health care today. Identifying priority content is best accomplished by nursing faculty who have expertise in the content they seek to teach. It is helpful to develop a list of questions that the textbook content should address and clearly answer. As an example, Table 8.2 shows a content checklist for evaluating psychiatric nursing texts.

TABLE 8.2 Content Checklist

Psychiatric/Mental Health Nursing Text

Diagnosis-related content:

_____Affective disorders

_____Bipolar disorder

_____Major depression

_____Anxiety disorders

_____Acute

_____Chronic

_____Death and dying

_____Dissociative disorders

_____Grief

_____Organic mental disorders

_____Paranoid disorder

_____Personality disorders

_____Antisocial personality

_____Borderline personality

_____Psychosis

_____Acute

_____Schizophrenia

_____Self-destructive behavior

_____Sexual dysfunction

_____Substance abuse

_____Violent behavior

_____Victims of violence

_____Violent clients

Contributory content:

_____Community mental health

_____Crisis intervention

_____Family components

_____Historical perspectives

_____Legal and ethical issues

_____Life-span considerations

(continued)

TABLE 8.2 Content Checklist *(continued)*

_____Psychoactive drugs

_____Psychosocial development

_____Research

_____Social and cultural aspects

_____Therapeutic approaches

    _____Alternative therapies

    _____Traditional therapies

_____Therapeutic groups

_____Therapeutic interpersonal communication

Other content included:

If more than one faculty member is evaluating the books for possible adoption, prepare the evaluation criteria together. Decide ahead of time how differences of opinion will be resolved about which book to adopt. Following the evaluation of the textbooks, share your evaluations and decide on the textbooks that will be adopted.

Date of Publication

Although date of publication is a factor to consider, some books are better even if they are a few years older than the ones that have been more recently published. Depending upon the editorial policies of a given book publisher or journal, what is in print may have been written from 1 to 3 years earlier. Because the lag time from writing to publishing is usually greater for books than for journals, what appears in journals may be more current or accurate. However, digital technology and online publishing have enabled textbooks to be more up to date and comprehensive than ever before.

For most textbooks, the publication (copyright) date is easy to find. If there is more than one date listed on the copyright page, the book has more than one edition. You can assume that most of the book was written at the time of the first date of publication, although new information may have been added in subsequent editions.

Cost

Textbook affordability has become an increasingly visible issue for college students, who have reported that the prices of textbooks are unexpected and staggering. According to the Federal Government

Accountability Office, textbook costs are now rising at almost four times the rate of inflation, and can average $900.00 for a single semester. For some community-college students, textbook expenses can comprise 40% of their total educational costs. Some publishers sell no-frill textbooks that have been printed inexpensively (color free, for example) with prices less than half of the higher quality colored-print textbook cost.

Faculty must know the costs of the textbooks they are reviewing for their courses, and cost should be an important consideration in textbook selection. If choosing between two or more texts that are about equal, choose the least expensive book. If the book is available in a less-expensive paperback version, ensure that the bookstore orders that format.

College Textbook Affordability Act

As of July 1, 2010, a new federal law, the College Textbook Affordability Act, aims to make textbooks more affordable for college students. The law, which was included in the Higher Education Act Reauthorization, is considered the first major federal action to address the climbing costs of textbooks for college students. This law requires textbook publishers to provide faculty with information regarding prices, formats (i.e., hardcover, paperback, online), revision plans, and differences between newer and older editions when they are making their sales pitch to faculty. The law also requires publishers to unbundle textbooks from CDs, workbooks, and other add-on items that hike the price, and may or may not be useful to students. With this information, faculty will be better able to select the most appropriate and least expensive options for their students.

In addition, the College Textbook Affordability Act requires faculty to provide students with textbook ISBN numbers, the name of the author, title, and date of publication of all required and optional course materials upon course registration. With this information, students will be able to determine book costs early and shop for the lowest available price.

Different Versions

Some authors have more than one version of their work. For example, Polit and Beck are both authors of *Essentials of Nursing Research* and *Nursing Research*. The first book is intended for consumers of nursing research, such as undergraduates, and the other book, written with Hungler, is for producers of research, such as graduate students.

Although not published by the same authors, there are books within each specialty area of nursing that are intended for one level of student or another. Hockenberry, Wilson, Winkelstein, and Kline have published *Wong's Nursing Care of Infants and Children,* while Whaley and Wong have published *Essentials of Pediatric Nursing.* The former is comprehensive and is intended for baccalaureate programs. The latter is more appropriate to associate-degree programs. Make sure to select the right book when you begin the evaluation process.

Electronic Textbooks (E-books)

Electronic textbooks, also known as e-books or digital textbooks, are becoming an alternative to traditional textbooks. E-books are the replication of traditional textbooks in digital format that can be read on a standard desktop or laptop computer screen, a PDA, or other portable device (e.g., Kindle e-readers), or on e-book applications through mobile devices (iPad, Android, Blackberry, iPhone). While e-books use many different file formats, most commonly PDF, they all share certain characteristics: They are portable, transferable, and searchable. E-books can also incorporate other features, such as annotations, audio and video files, and hyperlinks. E-books can include commenting and chat tools that allow interaction among readers, and some let users add links to external resources. Some e-book projects are tied to proprietary software, while others provide e-books in formats such as HTML.

E-Book Suppliers

E-books are sold at campus bookstores alongside printed texts. E-books are also made available to students through publishers' Web sites. CourseSmart (CourseSmart.com), a venture founded in 2007 by six higher education textbook publishers, is one of the largest distributors of e-books, with more than 12,500 textbook titles available by subscription.

School libraries can acquire e-books directly from publishers, distributors, or content aggregators and treat them as another information resource integrated into the online public access catalog (OPAC). Many times, colleges and university libraries will post their e-book holdings on their library home page as a drop-down menu categorized by academic programs.

Advantages of E-books

Faculty should be aware that the benefits of using e-books include lower costs than traditional textbooks (approximately 50% less than the retail price of a new hard copy textbook), and students have any-time access to reading assignments (via their laptop or portable device). In addition, e-book publishers can issue new editions on much shorter cycles, with some e-books updated annually. Some students prefer e-books because it lessens the physical load of books they carry.

Disadvantages of E-books

The disadvantages of e-books include publisher restrictions that may limit the number of devices that the e-textbook can be read on and how much of the text can be printed, shared, and copied/pasted. In addition, some publishers limit students' access to an e-book to one academic term, preventing the student from using the e-book as a future reference. Faculty should recognize that recent studies show that many students dislike e-books; students report that it is tiring to read on a digital screen for long periods of time and they prefer holding a traditional textbook.

Amount of Use

When selecting a book, ascertaining the proportion of the book you will actually use is important. If you can assign at least 60% to 75%, it is probably reasonable to consider the book. However, if there are many chapters that will not be assigned and that probably will not be assigned by other faculty in the program, it may be unreasonable to require students to purchase it.

If the program has more than one course with similar content, the same type of text may be required. For example, students may have a course dealing with fundamental medical-surgical nursing early in the program, whereas they have another course later dealing with complex medical-surgical content. If the two courses require the same kind of text, the faculty involved in the courses should collaborate on selecting texts. It may be necessary to have two different books, such as a text on fundamentals and a more comprehensive medical-surgical text. However, if the students are going to use the comprehensive type of text in both courses, the faculty should agree on one text rather than requiring the students to invest in two books with the same content.

Open-Access Textbooks

Some faculty members are beginning to experiment with freely available and licensed library materials as a substitute for textbooks. Although limited, there is a growing list of Web sites that allow free access to online textbooks, such as www.e-book.com.au/freebooks.htm.

Supplementing With Journal Readings

Because nursing students are making an investment in their textbooks, faculty should use textbooks as much as possible to satisfy the reading requirements for the class. However, many times supplemental journal readings are assigned to reinforce the central concepts addressed in the textbook or to provide current and in-depth perspectives on specific topics.

Although theory and lecture are appropriate to introduce cultural issues, many times faculty is limited in the application of those skills by the kinds of clinical experiences and patient populations their students experience. Journal articles can be a rich source of information on how cultural, ethnic, and religious practices impact health. Educators often use journal articles to integrate cultural content and experiences into the nursing curriculum, thereby developing culturally competent nursing students (Halloran, 2009).

In the event that a textbook is not available for a particular course, faculty must be cautious to choose the appropriate number of articles with content that makes up whole rather than fragmented parts. The details of weighing text and journal assignments are covered in the next section.

Journal Selection and Evaluation

Journal Sources

"Mapping the Nursing Literature Project," a recent study sponsored by the Nursing and Allied Health Resources (NAHRS) of the Medical

Library Association showed that the Cumulative Index to Nursing & Allied Health (CINAHL) provides the best coverage of nursing literature, followed by PubMed/MEDLINE, and then EBSCO Nursing & Allied Health Comprehensive Edition (Allen, Allison, & Stevens, 2006). The CINAHL database includes indexing for over 3,000 journals, including virtually all English-language nursing journals along with selected journals in 17 other allied health disciplines. Full text is available for more than 500 journals. CINAHL provides some journals that date back as early as 1937, and since the 1980s, CINAHL is updated monthly. In addition to journals, CINAHL includes health care books, nursing dissertations, selected conference proceedings, standards of professional practice, and educational software.

Accessibility to Journal Articles

Most faculty can assist students to access journal articles by using persistent links from their library's electronic resources. *Persistent links,* also called *durable links* or *bookmarks,* are Internet addresses that connect directly to specific full-text articles. Most persistent links can be placed within course management system (i.e., Coursework, Blackboard) class sites, syllabi, and reading lists.

A word of caution: A few journals do not allow their persistent links to be used in online syllabi or course management systems. Such use restrictions will always be stated at the end of the full-text article.

Although some publishers allow journal articles to be posted in entirety as a PDF on the course management system, using a persistent link is always preferable because a publisher's policy can change and your institution could risk high fines for violation of copyright. Additionally, using a persistent link acquaints students with library resources and allows the library to evaluate databases through usage reports.

It is important to copy the persistent link from the article record rather than the URL appearing in the browser address bar, which is temporary and may not work later on. For some databases, you will need to add the library proxy prefix to the beginning of the persistent link so that students can be authenticated to access the article when they are off campus. Always test a persistent link before saving it in your course management system.

Primarily because of financial constraints, many university and college libraries have a limited number of journals that are available electronically. Nursing faculty should carefully identify the journals that they rely on and commonly reference for reading assignments. In doing so, faculty can encourage librarians to add journal titles to their annual purchases of electronic media.

Journal Articles Available Online in Open Access

Some journal articles may be available for free via open-access Web sites. These open-access publications can be found in university repositories or in open-access journals. For the most part, open-access journals can be posted on your course management systems without problems. A word of caution: Although the price is right for free/open Web sites, they require Internet access, may require printing, and if they vanish from the Internet, oh well.

Bio Med Central (BMC) Nursing is an open-access journal, publishing original peer-reviewed research articles in all aspects of nursing research, training, education, and practice. BMC Nursing (ISSN 1472–6955) is indexed/tracked/covered by PubMed, CAS, EMBASE, Scopus, CINAHL and Google Scholar. BMC Nursing can be accessed at http://www.biomedcentral.com/bmcnurs/.

The Directory of Open Access Journals (DOAJ) is a Web-based service that covers free, full-text, quality-controlled scientific and scholarly journals. Access DOAJ at www.doaj.org.

The OAIster® database (www.oaister.worldcat.org) offers millions of free digital resources from thousands of libraries worldwide.

Global Nursing Knowledge Network offers nursing scholarly articles free (http://www.gnkn.org/).

Although PubMed finds articles that are not open access, if you select the "Limits" tab and check "Links to full free text," the search will produce only those articles that are open access to all. To reach the article from the list, click on links opposite the title, click on LINK OUT, and then follow the directions (http://www.ncbi.nlm.nih.gov/entrez/).

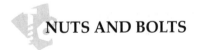

NUTS AND BOLTS

Procedures for Textbook Review

Identifying Potential Textbooks

There are a number of ways that faculty members identify potential textbooks in both traditional print and digital formats (electronic books). Faculty find out about textbooks from publishers' ads in journals and other media, book reviews in journals, contacts with publishers' representatives on campus or at meetings, and contacts with colleagues. Publishers may provide email alerts to their mailing lists regarding topics of interest. Faculty can write to the publishers of nursing texts and ask to be put on their mailing and email lists for catalogues and other book announcements. Browsing the publisher's Web sites is another easy way to identify potential texts.

An efficient way to identify potential e-books is through the R2 Digital Library. Faculty should check with their librarian to see if the college or university subscribes to the R2 Digital Library, a Web-based database available from Rittenhouse Book Distributors. Using the R2 Digital Library allows faculty to search medical, nursing, and allied health source-book content from key health science publishers on a Web-based platform. Content is available from publishers such as Lippincott Williams & Wilkins, The McGraw-Hill Companies, The American Academy of Pediatrics, and many more. In addition, the R2 Digital Library has many features that are valuable to users, such as customized saved searches, images, references and bookmarks, an A-Z Drug Index, and an A-Z Topic Index. Access at the R2 Digital Library at http://www.r2library.com/public/default.aspx.

Some publishers are now making it easy for faculty to develop custom textbooks by picking and choosing chapters and customizing tables of contents. Custom books help ensure that students only pay for what they need for the course.

Securing Textbooks for Review

Some publishers will automatically send a new edition of a book that has been adopted for a class. Sales representatives will call or visit the school to get lists of the faculty members and their specialties. Faculty who want a specific book can get review copies of texts by calling or writing to the publisher of the book. Use their response cards for this or write on the letterhead of the school. Publishers usually want to know the name of the course, how many times a year the course is offered, and the average enrollment of students. They also may want to know what book you currently use, who will participate in the selection, and when a decision will be made. Usually, it is possible to get a complimentary copy of a text that can be kept whether or not the book is adopted. If it is a specialty book that is not usually used as a text, faculty may only be able to review it for a set time if it is not adopted. If the text is adopted, faculty will probably be able to keep it without charge.

Review Timetable

Set a specific time period during which textbooks will be reviewed for adoption, or review them on an ongoing basis. Many texts are published in the early part of the year so as to be hot off the press when faculty are making their decisions for the coming academic year. Be sure there is time enough for the bookstore to be able to get the copies for the students. Sometimes a book is so well received that distributors run out of copies, and the bookstore may not be able to get them until after the term starts.

Rules of Thumb in Assigning Textbook and Journal Reading Assignments

Read the Assigned Reading

Taking the time to read the assigned readings carefully is a simple but vital task. If a chapter in a text or an article contains certain terms in its title, sometimes it is taken for granted that the topic of those terms is covered adequately. However, the piece may have one of the following shortcomings:

It neglects important points.
It does not emphasize priorities.
It includes too much detail.
It repeats or contradicts other readings.

Amount of Reading

Faculty members must have reasonable expectations concerning the length and difficulty of reading assignments. It is important to recognize that the quality of the reading assignment is more important than the quantity. A rule of thumb for assignments to be completed outside of class is to allow for 2 to 3 hours of reading per week per credit hour. For example, 2 hours x 3 credits = 6 hours/week of outside work.

Accessibility

Obviously, assignments from the students' textbooks will be the most accessible. When readings are assigned outside the students' texts, consider how available these will be. Although it is legitimate to want to encourage students to use the library, there may be better ways to accomplish that goal than to require them to go to the library when their texts will suffice.

Evaluate the holdings and the policies of the library the students will use. If you will be providing your own copy of a book or article, find out how the library handles these materials. If you provide photo-copied material, make sure that copyright laws are followed.

Copyright

Reproduction of copyrighted material without prior permission of the copyright owner is an issue for the academic community. Remember: As in other applications of the law, "Ignorance is no defense." As an educator, there is an expectation to understand the copyright law to indulge only in fair use of copied material. To begin with, indiscriminate copying of published works deprives authors of control of their written work as well as income. Although the law is somewhat generous to teachers as to what constitutes fair use, it is important that all aspects of the law are followed. It is essential that all faculty members have a copy of *Questions and Answers on Copyright for the Campus Community*, which is published by the National Association of College Stores, the Association of American Publishers, and the Association of American University Presses.

Some publishers of journals sell reprints of articles expected to be of continuing use. They are not likely to give permission to make copies. In this situation, request that the library or the administration purchase reprints, or make this a required purchase the students will make when they buy their textbooks. The U.S. Library of Congress provides a comprehensive document, *Circular 21: Reproduction of Copyrighted Works by Educators and Librarians*, which can be accessed at http://www.copyright.gov/circs/circ21.pdf.

Unique Contribution

Faculty members should avoid assigning repetitious material when they choose assignments. They sometimes assign a three- or four-page article when only a small portion conveys something different or in addition to other reading available in the text.

Contradictions

Another reason to read the assignments before the students is to validate that they are in harmony with one another. If there are real or apparent contradictions between readings, clarify for students which account is the one they need to learn, or help them to understand that there are differences of opinion on the issue.

FINAL WORDS

Good teachers know that it takes time, a lot of work, and thought to choose the best readings for their students. Selecting the most appropriate textbooks and reading assignments is a key activity in teaching effectively. Textbook and journal reading assignments should provide students correct, credible, and up-to-date information. Moreover, textbooks and reading assignments should foster critical thinking, critical reflection, cultural competence, and evidence-based practice. When selecting textbooks and reading assignments, faculty should identify the learning needs of their students. Because most undergraduate nursing students today are millennial learners, carefully consider the need for electronic textbooks and reading assignments that are delivered with interactive, digital, and multimedia technologies. In doing so, faculty will learn how to use these innovative technologies to teach, inspire, and develop their nursing students.

FURTHER READING

Allen, M., Allison, M. M., & Stevens, S. (2006). Mapping the literature of nursing education. *The Journal of Medical Library Associations, 94*(2), e122–e127.

Cassata, L. C., & Cox, T. M. (2009). Evaluation tool for clinical nursing textbooks: Bridging content analysis and evidence. *The Journal of Nursing Education, 48*(6), 301–309.

Fitzpatrick, J. (2008). If my syllabus could talk: What would it say about me? *Nursing Education Perspectives, 29*, 1, 5.

Halloran, L. (2009). Teaching transcultural nursing through literature. *Journal of Nursing Education, 48*(9), 523–528. doi:10.3928/ 01484834–20090610–07

Hernon, P., Hopper, R., Leach, M. R., Saunders, L. L., & Zhang, J. (2006). E-books use by students: Undergraduates in economics, literature, and nursing. *The Journal of Academic Leadership, 33*(1), 3–13.

Library of Congress Copyright Office. (2009). *Reproduction of copyrighted works by educators and librarians.* Washington, DC. Retrieved from http://www.copyright.gov/circs/circ21.pdf

Mangold, K. (2007). Educating a new generation: Teaching baby boomer faculty about millennial students. *Nurse Educator, 32*, 21–23.

McCurry, M., & Martins, D. C. (2010). Teaching undergraduate nursing research: A comparison of traditional and innovative approaches for success with millennial learners. *Journal of Nursing Education, 49*(5), 276–279. doi:10.3928/01484834–20091217–02

Oermann, M. H., & Christman, J. (2008). Reading assignments in nursing courses: Some guidelines for faculty. *Teaching and Learning in Nursing, 3*, 56–58.

9

Designing and Grading a Major Assignment

Grading assignments is a time-consuming part of a faculty member's work. Have you ever stopped to think about giving assignments? What do you as faculty hope to gain from them? What do students get from doing assignments? Ideally, an assignment will enhance learning. Some students seem frustrated and overwhelmed by any assignment, but hopefully the assignments will be challenging for those who can handle them yet manageable for those who are not up to the challenge.

An assignment should fit within the context of the course, especially in terms of the course objectives. For example, an assignment would not be appropriate in a lower division course, with primarily lower cognitive levels of objectives, which can be met by listening to lectures, viewing media, and reading. Because it is typical for upper division and graduate courses to have higher level objectives, students in those courses need experiences exceeding those in lower division courses. It is helpful in evaluating students to give them assignments that permit them to demonstrate higher order cognitive skills.

GOALS

A major assignment should be used to allow the student to demonstrate accomplishment of high-level objectives. Such an assignment permits the evaluation of learning, which is not easily evaluated objectively.

DEFINITION OF A MAJOR ASSIGNMENT

The qualities that differentiate between major and minor assignments are (1) the depth and breadth of the content involved, (2) the time required for completion, and (3) the amount of credit attached to the evaluation of the finished product. When any of these qualities is substantial, the assignment is defined as major.

One determination of substantive work involved in fulfilling an assignment is the amount of work required outside of class. A general rule for determining a reasonable amount of work outside of class is a ratio of 2 or 3 hours to each hour spent in class. A formula for calculating amount of work outside of class would be credit hours × 2 (or 3) hours × weeks in quarter or semester.

The calculation for a three-credit semester course is 3 × 2 (or 3) × 15 = 90 (or 135) hours outside of class. This outside work would include all the required reading and the preparation of assignments necessary for the student to meet the requirements of the course. If a great deal of reading were required, the time remaining to devote to an assignment would be limited. By the same token, a major assignment would limit the time for outside reading.

A major assignment is usually designed to give students an opportunity to choose one thing to study to a greater extent, either in terms of increased depth, breadth, or both. For example, in a graduate course on nursing theory, students might be assigned to study one theory in depth. In an undergraduate course, students might be given an assignment to identify 10 different interventions to reach the same outcome.

The amount of work involved should be directly related to the portion of the course grade to be determined by the grade on the assignment. For example, an assignment that will take one-third of the allotted time outside of class to complete could be rewarded with a major portion of the course grade.

TYPES OF ASSIGNMENTS

Major Paper

Purposes

A major paper, usually 10 to 12 pages, not only allows students to demonstrate abilities with higher cognitive objectives but also permits them the opportunity to practice putting their ideas in writing. A paper is particularly useful when your aims relate to critical thinking, analysis, or organizational skills.

Preparation

The time that is required for students to prepare a paper might be extensive, depending on your expectations. There are two different approaches to determining the content requirements of the paper. A student-centered paper includes a description or analysis of something the student did, as with nursing care plans. The other major type of paper is concept centered, in which the student investigates a concept or issue in depth, such as a paper on a professional issue or a physiological or psychosocial principle. A paper based on the student's own activities usually requires less time in gathering information but more time in organizing and analyzing. A paper dealing with a concept or issue requires more investigation of the literature and also calls for organization and analysis.

The complexity of a paper is related to the extent of the literature search required to support the student's ideas. It takes time for the student to locate appropriate resources and read the selections. For students less experienced with the process of writing a paper, each reference might take up to 3 hours to locate, read, and incorporate into the paper. Students who have had experience have often learned ways of simplifying some of these steps, but it is a good idea to assess their abilities in this regard. This process is dealt with at greater length in Chapter 14.

Although it varies, depending upon the complexity of the ideas involved, an average student may take an hour or more to compose one page of text. If the student is conscientious in writing, there will be at least one or two drafts before the final copy. This means it could take a student between 10 and 20 hours to compose a 10-page paper, apart from the literature search and reading time.

Grading

Develop a list of evaluation criteria such as those in Table 9.1 and use it as a grading guide. To increase objectivity, some faculty prefer to use a rubric format for grading, especially if there are multiple faculty members and teaching assistants grading the course papers. A scoring rubric contains details of the criteria for the paper and has grade points allocated for each criterion. Rubric-generating software is available and provides good

TABLE 9.1   Evaluation Criteria for a Major Paper

Assessment	
Data are logically summarized	5
Significant data are identified	5
Planning	
State appropriate outcomes	15
Identify three top priorities	10
State criteria for evaluation of outcomes	10
Implementation	
Identify interventions to accomplish the three top priorities for care	20
Cite references for interventions	10
Describe one unique intervention	5
Evaluation	
Evaluate outcomes for three top priorities	5
Evaluate own performance of care	5
Style and format	
Paper is typewritten and double spaced	3
APA form is used for references	3
Correct grammar and spelling are used	4
Total points	100

language for descriptors for each cell in the rubric. A sample of a rubric is in Table 9.2. Objectivity in grading is important, but even so there will always be a certain degree of subjectivity. It may be beneficial to share the evaluation criteria or rubric with the students before they write the paper. This will help the students with the paper outline and let them know where to put the most time and effort when writing the paper.

Major papers take a long time to grade, and nursing students often concentrate on getting the assignment done rather than spending time trying to make what they write interesting. Because of this, carefully consider whether a major paper is appropriate for the course requirements. If this will be a valuable way to assess students' achievement of objectives, be sure to have the papers submitted in time to allow plenty of time for grading.

Experienced faculty members know that the worst papers take the most time to grade. The sentence structure, grammar, and organization may be difficult to follow. Some students have difficulty with what

TABLE 9.2   Sample of a Grading Rubric

	5 Excellent	4 Very good	3 Average	2 Below average	1 Unsatisfactory
Content					
Meeting objectives					
Accurate current information					
Appropriate coverage of information					
Examples relating to content					
Content Total =					
Process					
Introduction					
Organization					
Quality of Grammar (if rubric is for paper)					
Summary					
Process Total =					
Total Grade = _____ (Content + Process)					

content they should include, no matter how clearly it was described in the requirements.

Students who did poorly on the paper will probably feel they spent a lot of time on it and that they should get a better grade simply because of the amount of time involved. Never doubt the time students claim they spend, but point out to them that the product is what they are being graded on.

Occasionally, a student will submit a paper that is exceptional because it is thoughtfully done and well written. However, that does not happen as often as one would like.

Projects

Purposes

A project offers the opportunity for application of knowledge in a practical situation. Some examples familiar to nursing educators are community studies, teaching projects, health screening, research critiques, and research proposals. Although such assignments may be done outside of class, in some cases they may be done during clinical time.

Preparation

Although a project may be completed within the allotted course time, the requirements may necessitate students' completing some work outside of the scheduled time. Faculty must spend time orienting and supervising students involved in projects, especially because they generally include some contact with people outside the educational program. Give the students ground rules for making outside contacts. For example, students completing a community assessment should have proper identification such as a student ID to show to people they want to interview. They should have appropriate data-collection tools if they are asking people for information to assess health needs.

Supervising

A project may require indirect supervision by faculty. Schedule periodic meetings with students to ascertain their progress and to monitor their performance. The supervisory meetings are also useful for teaching the processes involved in the project. For example, students completing a community study need instruction as they proceed through the steps involved, just as they do in learning how to take care of individuals in the hospital.

Appropriate supervision requires significant amounts of time. Undergraduate students need structure to meet the expectations of supervision. It is helpful to post a sign-up sheet with meeting times specified. This makes faculty availability to students apparent. If periodic meetings are required over the semester to discuss project work, designate the weeks in which the students must sign up. Email may be an appropriate way to make appointments and also to discuss assignments with busy students. Part of the role as a faculty member is determining when it is appropriate to make decisions or to introduce structure. With undergraduates, a lot of time is wasted unnecessarily by expecting the students to make decisions they have not learned how to make.

Grading

Projects are time consuming to grade. Some are best graded by observing students in the process of fulfilling the work, such as in doing health screening. Given the conditions under which such an event may occur, it is usually difficult to discriminate between various levels of performance. In such situations, rather than specific interactions, evaluate the planning and overall implementation to assess the safety of and respect for the client.

Other projects may require the production of a written work to be graded. As with papers, any written work is time consuming to grade. Because the emphasis in assigning a project is on application, written materials should be graded with that in mind. In other words, there should be less emphasis on style and form unless they are indicated within the context of your course.

Presentations

Purpose

A presentation gives students the opportunity to share their work. It gives them the chance to organize information for an activity that is more common for most nurses than are written forms of presentation.

Preparation

Orienting students to a presentation is similar to giving guidelines for a paper. Tell them the parameters so that they can achieve the objectives. These are further discussed in the next major section. Some faculty members incorrectly see this format as an easy way to put on a course. Facilitating the experience of the students enrolled in a course is the responsibility of faculty. Be prepared to help correct misconceptions when students make mistakes in factual data and to help the entire group relate the material presented to the course as a whole.

Grading

A presentation is fairly easy to grade if there is a checklist based on the criteria that were set in advance. It is best used at the time of the presentation. In some instances, there is value in having part of the evaluation done by the other members of the class, as well as by the faculty member and the presenter. If students are going to be evaluating each other and themselves, establish ground rules such as sticking to the criteria, using objective comments, describing specific behaviors, and using care in expressing negative opinions. A sample checklist is shown in Table 9.3.

Combinations of Assignments

Frequently, students are asked to combine two or three assignments. Whenever a second or third dimension is added to the assignment, there

TABLE 9.3 Checklist for Grading Presentations

The following scale is used for the evaluation:

    5 = Excellent
    4 = Very good
    3 = Average
    2 = Below average
    1 = Unsatisfactory

Content:

Meeting objectives	1	2	3	4	5
Accurate, current information	1	2	3	4	5
Appropriate coverage of information	1	2	3	4	5
Examples relating to content	1	2	3	4	5

Process:

Introduction	1	2	3	4	5
Organization	1	2	3	4	5
Quality of grammar, pronunciation	1	2	3	4	5
Summary	1	2	3	4	5

Scores

Content	_____	17–20 = A
Process	_____	11–16 = B
Total	_____	7–12 = C
Average	_____	5–8 = D
		<5 = F

is a need to consider the extra work required along with the expectations for each dimension. Decide how much credit will be attached to each part while keeping in mind the basic objectives of the original assignment. For example, if a project is involved and if it takes a lot of time, most of the credit given should be attached to the portion requiring the most work. Some students might implement their projects well but do poorly in the class presentation. They should not be penalized on the presentation if the principal objectives were met by what the students did well.

TOOLS

Designing the Assignment

Start by describing the assignment in a brief, concise manner, using straightforward language. It is important to have a clear purpose for the assignment. Next, list the objectives to be accomplished by the student in the completion of the assignment. A sample description and objectives are given in Table 9.4.

TABLE 9.4   Assignment Description and Objectives

Nursing Care Study

The student will write a paper describing the nursing care of one patient. The paper will focus on the student's care giving only. All steps of the nursing process are to be discussed with emphasis on the planning and implementation steps. Prior to beginning the paper, the student must have the selected patient approved by the clinical instructor who will grade the paper.

The objectives to be met by the student are as follows:

1. Summarize data collection and identify significant data points for nursing intervention.
2. Demonstrate ability to set appropriate outcomes for the patient.
3. Identify the top three priorities in the patient's care.
4. Describe measurable criteria for evaluating outcomes.
5. Describe nursing interventions that relate to the identified priorities.
6. Use theoretical references to support nursing.
7. Devise at least one unique intervention.
8. Evaluate nursing care outcomes using criteria.
9. Evaluate own performance of nursing care.
10. Use established standards for the preparation of a written paper.

Required Content and Format

Although the description and objectives indicate the content, restate what is to be emphasized in the assignment. In the example given in Table 9.4, it might be helpful to stress that the focus is on two particular steps in the nursing process, although the student is to demonstrate some attention to the other two.

Supply undergraduates with a specific format to follow; for example, give them a specific outline. The outline or format can be useful for projects, papers, or presentations and helps to ensure that the students fulfill the requirements. A sample of a format is given in Table 9.5.

Include format stipulations about the use of references if these are appropriate. Designate the parameters in terms of how recent the references should be or what would be acceptable resources.

TABLE 9.5   Format for a Paper

Nursing Care Study

Content

The study is to be in narrative form. Use the following major headings for the organization of the content.

Introduction: Describe the patient briefly.

Data Collection: Summarize the data collected on the patient and list the significant data on which your study will focus.

Outcome: State the outcome objectives you set.

Evaluation Criteria: Describe the criteria by which you planned to determine your success in meeting outcome objectives.

Priorities: List the top three priorities for care, and support your selection with references and data.

Interventions: Describe the interventions used for each objective, including references for their use. At least one intervention should be unique.

Evaluation: Using your evaluation criteria, describe how the patient met or did not meet those criteria. Evaluate your ability to perform the necessary nursing care using appropriate course objectives.

Summary: Summarize your role in the care of the patient.

Grading the Assignment

Criteria for Evaluation

Base the criteria on the objectives, and state them clearly. Specify in advance how the points will be assigned to each part of the assignment. Identifying such criteria gives the student information about the requirements for each portion of the assignment. They help the student know the depth and breadth of information required for each section prior to doing the assignment. Examples are given in Tables 9.1 and 9.2 earlier in this chapter.

Submission Requirements

Clearly specify submission or completion requirements. When any written work is part of the assignment, encourage or require students to make a copy of their work before submitting the original for evaluation. With written work, set a submission date with some stipulation about how late submissions will be handled. If extensions are given without penalties for certain reasons, identify these exceptions. For example, illness or family emergencies may warrant an extension. Assess a reasonable penalty for late submissions based on the value of the assignment and the real inconvenience a late paper may cause. For example, assess a penalty of one to five points for each day the paper is late. Be sure to stipulate if weekends are or are not counted in the days late. Give clear instructions regarding acceptable methods of submission of completed assignments, for example, electronic submissions.

If the assignment is a presentation, set the date for the presentation as far in advance as possible. Let the students know how much time will be available for the presentation so they can plan accordingly. Make clear the criteria for evaluation of the presentation. Often, presentations are evaluated in terms of process as well as content. Establish clear ground rules about the relative weights of such grades and make the tool for the evaluation available to the students in advance. Have a plan in mind as to what to do with class time if the student or students scheduled to present are unable to do so.

If the assignment is a project, go over the requirements in detail with the students before they get started, and plan one or two meetings with the individuals or groups involved. Usually, a project is completed by submitting a written paper or by giving a presentation. This will make the submission criteria more complex. Bear in mind what the original purpose of the project was when evaluating the form in which it is reported.

Plagiarism

In this digital era there is a growing problem with plagiarism; that is, when a writer takes another writer's information, words, or ideas and uses it as his or her own. Much plagiarism is accidental, such as when students unintentionally cite and reference sources incorrectly. Faculty members usually have to spend time teaching students how to use a writing style guide such as the *Publication Manual of the American Psychological Association* (APA, 2009). Daggett (2008) designed a very useful rubric for grading the APA aspects of a paper. If you plan to use this rubric, make sure you are using the most recent APA guidelines. Sharing a rubric like this or a sample paper with all the common APA elements will help the students use APA style correctly. Detecting plagiarism can be difficult. Here are a few things you can look for as you read a student's paper. Are there sections of the paper that have a very different writing style from the rest of the paper? Is the content of the paper at a much higher standard than other work the student has produced? If the answer is yes to either of these questions, you can take a portion of the paper under examination and place it in an Internet search engine. You may find that the whole section used in the paper appears in the search results. Also, there are a number of plagiarism-detection software programs available, such as Turnitin. In some schools of nursing, all student papers are screened using this software before they are graded. The papers must be submitted electronically in order for them to be screened. If you are using a plagiarism-detection program, let your students know, as it will heighten their awareness of the seriousness of plagiarism. Also, remind students of the academic integrity policies in the school of nursing and the academic institutions.

INDIVIDUAL AND GROUP ASSIGNMENTS

Many assignments are made for individuals to complete. Because the kind of assignment being discussed here is often oriented toward synthesis and other high-level processes, evaluation of each person's ability to demonstrate these skills is important. Even if some of these skills may eventually be used as part of a team, each person knowing something about each step in a process is beneficial. Although this may result in a superficial treatment of some aspects of the assignment, at least each individual comes out of it with some knowledge about each part.

Individual assignments and individual evaluations are particularly appropriate in three situations. The first is when the assignment is something usually undertaken and accomplished by a single person in actual practice. The second circumstance is when an assignment is manageable for one person to complete in the amount of time you have allotted. The final situation is one in which it is important for each student to accomplish and demonstrate the skills involved.

Some major assignments are complex enough that group work is necessary to fulfill the requirements. For example, a community assessment is extremely complex if done thoroughly. For such an activity, students may learn more responsibility by focusing on a part of the assignment and by sharing the responsibility.

For other assignments, a group effort may more closely simulate what happens in actual practice or convey a philosophical stance on how an activity should be carried out. A good example of this is a research proposal or project. Although a great deal of nursing research has been attempted by individuals, a good many expert nurse researchers emphasize the worth of nurses doing more research in small teams. By making projects group assignments, students see the value of this approach.

Individual assignments are more time consuming to grade than are a smaller number of group projects. Instead of grading 20 individual papers, you might have six or eight group projects.

Supervising and evaluating group work is more complex than working with individuals. Problems frequently occur due to difficulty within groups in working out individual responsibilities for the overall assignment. This can be partially remedied by meeting with the groups and helping them to establish their own ground rules. After all, if part of the intent is for them to learn how to work in a group, students need guidance on this as well as in dealing with the content itself. Before making the assignment a group activity, give some thought to how the groups can present their final product so that assessment of individual achievement is possible.

Decide how to handle grievances over allegations by group members that others in the group are not taking their share of responsibility. For example, if one person seems not to be doing his or her work, what proof would you require of this? How would you deal with it if it were proved to you? Getting caught in the middle of this kind of situation is pretty uncomfortable.

Support all the students and help them to establish some ground rules to deal with the identified problem. Often the students who originally complained are as much at fault as the one they are complaining about.

One way to avoid this type of situation is to have frequent meetings with the groups. Their ability to work as a group in such meetings will reflect how they are doing when the group works alone. The supervision of group work is discussed in more detail in Chapter 4.

FINAL WORDS

Major assignments help evaluate students' abilities to accomplish high-level objectives. Spend time in the design of the assignment requirements and criteria for evaluation to ensure a successful outcome. As with other teaching tools, putting effort in the design of assignments will make them more manageable for you to evaluate.

FURTHER READING

American Psychological Association. (2009). *Publication manual of the American Psychological Association* (6th ed.). Washington, DC: Author.

Caputi, L. (2006). Grading papers: Pleasure or pain? *Teaching and Learning in Nursing, 1*(2), 35–42. doi:10.1016/j.teln.2006.06.004

Daggett, L. (2008). A rubric for grading or editing student papers. *Nurse Educator, 33*(2), 55–56.

Freeman, S., & Parks, J. W. (2010). How accurate is peer grading? *CBE-Life Sciences Education, 9*(4), 482–488. doi:10.1187/cbe.10–03–0017

Holmes, V. (1997). Grading journals in clinical practice: A delicate issue. *Journal of Nursing Education, 36*(10), 489–492.

Rieck, S., & Crouch, L. (2007). Connectiveness and civility in online learning. *Nurse Education in Practice, 7*(6), 425–432. doi:10.1016/j.nepr.2007.06.006

10

Designing and Grading a Minor Assignment

A minor assignment is different from a major assignment in that it is less substantive in terms of depth and breadth of the content, requires less time for completion, and has less credit attached to the finished product. Generally, minor assignments are focused on something specific, such as on a short essay about a student's thoughts about an event or concept. Such assignments should take only an hour or two to complete. Minor assignments are particularly suitable in the clinical arena. The credit given for minor assignments is relatively small compared with other course requirements that call for more work. In some instances, credit may be given in a blanket manner, such as a requirement for four short essays. As long as they are submitted at the specified times, the student receives a certain amount of credit. The faculty member does not have to evaluate the quality of each essay, only note that each was submitted. Some assignments considered to be major in one context might be considered minor in another. For example, a critique of a research article would be a major assignment for the student initially learning about research. For graduate students, such a critique would be minor.

GOALS

Minor assignments are used to measure medium- to higher-level objectives. These assignments are useful methods to evaluate learning that is not easily measured by objective means.

TYPES OF MINOR ASSIGNMENTS

Short Essay

A short essay is about two to five typed pages. The content is focused on one objective or one incident. A short essay might, for example, describe a student's first reaction to a given clinical setting. There are few or no references required, with emphasis being placed on the student's ideas or involvement. The format is simple, perhaps including only an introduction, the body of the paper with no subtopics, and a conclusion. Grading short essays takes time, particularly if there are a large number of students. However, the advantage of the short essay is that the highest level of cognitive domain objectives, such as analysis, synthesis, and evaluation, can be tested.

Critique

A critique is a critical discussion. In nursing education, a critique is often done on the elements of a published research study. A critique helps to foster a student's appreciation of the parts of research. By using established criteria to evaluate a research study, a student learns to use critical thinking skills.

Students need guidelines to learn to do critiques. Most texts on nursing research provide useful outlines to give students the necessary structure. In an undergraduate research course, a critique may be a major assignment and might be done over many weeks as the students learn more about the research process. However, as a student advances, the process of doing critiques becomes part of more major assignments.

Students are evaluated on their ability to apply the relevant criteria correctly and to draw the appropriate kinds of conclusions. For students who are just learning about the process, requirements are less stringent. For more advanced students, it would be appropriate to expect them to recognize subtleties or sophisticated aspects of the process involved in doing the critique.

Journal Entry

A journal entry is short and might be completed in one page. It is specifically focused and briefly describes the student's position or ideas relating to an objective or event. The student may be asked to describe feelings about a particular topic or experience. Journal entries are often used in clinical and experiential learning experiences. The faculty member should provide the student with clear guidelines as to the objective, content, length, and due date of the journal entry. Journal entries can be submitted electronically using email or the drop box within a Web-based course-management system such as Blackboard. This type of assignment is personal, and the student's work is shared only with the faculty member. Journal entries are not usually graded, but a designated number of points out of the total grade are allocated for submission of journal entries. The faculty member is focused on reading about the student's reflection of the experience as well as providing an opportunity for improvement of writing skills. Timely feedback is important, particularly as the student's reflection of an experience will affect subsequent experiences, and so the faculty member may need to discuss the reflection further with the student. With online submission of the journal entry assignment, the faculty member can provide individual feedback more quickly to all students and invite further online discussion with students who will benefit from such discussion. Table 10.1 shows a sample journal entry.

TABLE 10.1   A Journal Entry

My Most Challenging Patient

My most challenging patient was a 23-year-old woman who was admitted with acute abdominal pain, diarrhea, and projectile vomiting. I had to start an IV, insert an NG tube, and give her an injection in preparation to go to surgery. It took at least 24 minutes to talk her into each procedure while she whined and verbally abused me for trying to do each thing.

The last thing I did before she went to OR was to help her with the bedpan. While I was cleaning it, she said, "I think you became a nurse just to make people suffer." I said, "I can see why you might feel that way, but I really want to help you." She said, "Ha!" I made sure the bed rails were secure and left.

When the aide came with the carrier to take her to OR, I went to help transfer her. When they started to wheel her away, she said, "I am so scared." I took her hand and said, "I will go with you." I held her hand until they took her into OR. The last thing she said to me was, "Thanks, nurse." I felt wonderful!

Response Paper

The purpose of a response paper is to ask students to respond to something in particular, usually a journal article. This assignment permits students to demonstrate critical thinking and encourages them to synthesize what they are reading. Students may be asked to identify applications of an article that is primarily theoretical, for example. As with other assignments, set more specific guidelines for students in undergraduate courses. If working with graduate students, the assignment may be open ended, and part of the expectation would be for students to identify their own focus for such an activity.

Often response papers are not graded, but faculty will assign a percentage of the course grade based on the effort involved. Overall the faculty member is focused on the student's writing skills and ability to the express thoughts in writing. Web-based course management systems' discussion boards or group pages may be used to facilitate the involvement of other students in this exercise. The faculty member could assign the same reading to all the students and ask them to post their responses on the class discussion board by a designated date. Then, after this date and within a short designated period (up to a week), each student must respond substantively to perhaps two of their colleagues' postings. By substantively, we mean about 250 words, not just "Nice posting, Rebecca." If there is a large number of students, the faculty member can divide the students into groups of four or five and set up a group discussion boards for each group. Then each person in the group has to respond to perhaps two of their colleagues' postings. This group method works well with large classes because the main disadvantage of a general class discussion board is that after the first few students have written their responses, the remaining students feel there is nothing new to add. Assessing the involvement of the other students involves assessing their writing skills and having the ability to critique the work of others. Again, the designated percentage of the course grade for a response paper will include this additional student effort. Each student will receive an individual grade.

Logs

A log may be kept on a weekly basis to deal with the interpersonal aspects of the clinical setting, service learning, or other experiential learning. Logs are probably more common assignments in psychiatric settings or community health nursing experiences. A log helps students to evaluate and incorporate their personal experiences in a situation uncommon to their usual activities.

Give students structure about the content and processes that are expected in the log. For example, ask them to take no more than one or two pages for each entry. In each entry, ask them to describe the most interesting thing that happened during the week, or ask them to discuss how a particular concept was applied or how a certain objective was met. This type of instruction will help the student to provide a useful log rather than just a log that keeps track of the hours and lists the experiences.

Logs may be given credit for simply being done and submitted as required rather than being graded. This is especially important if you are asking students to be honest and open about their own feelings— they should be given credit for doing so, but you can hardly grade feelings. It would be more appropriate to give encouraging comments, such as "You really opened up this week," or "This must have been tough for you." If the entry pertains to something factual or cognitive, you might say, "You did a good job of describing this situation," or "This is a good example of the concept." Logs can be submitted to faculty electronically. Again, timely faculty feedback will encourage students and facilitate student growth. One suggestion is to have the students keep their logs in the same document and to submit the complete document each time. This allows the faculty member to review the students' continuous progress easily.

Case Study

A case study is another example of a strategy for a minor assignment. The faculty member designs a case study keeping in mind the learning objectives and the level of the learner. Following the case study a series of questions are presented. These questions may involve identification of the patient's problem, decisions related to the patient's management, medication questions, short- and long-term care outcomes, and possible complications. These questions are the key component for the assignment and must be clear and related to the learning objectives.

A variation on the case study is the unfolding case study. The unfolding case study has the advantage of adding clinical information to the case study as it unfolds, thereby changing the scenario and increasing the complexity of the assignment. In an assignment with an unfolding case study, the faculty member may provide a case study followed by a series of questions. Once the student has responded to these questions, the next section is presented, which adds additional information that may have changed the student's previous responses. In the second section, the student is asked to state if this new information would change his or her clinical decisions for the case study patient, and if so, how.

Simulations

Simulations are student activities that reflect the clinical environment such as role play and the use of high-fidelity simulators—highly interactive computerized mannequins—that are used to teach critical thinking and psychomotor skills. If the faculty member plans to use the high-fidelity patient simulators, he or she will need to have skills necessary to design appropriate learning simulations (e.g., a patient scenario with unfolding events based on the student's actions), and then program the mannequin for the simulation experience. Technical support personnel are important in this process. These simulations provide life-like experiences for the student. For a successful learning experience, the faculty member will organize the students into small groups with a designated role for each student in the health care team. Simulation assignments can be designed for an individual student in the role of nurse, and other members of the group may be observers, a second nurse, the patient's relative, and so forth. Provide the ground rules and expectations for the simulation exercise with emphasis on the roles the students are playing. Throughout the simulation assignment the faculty member will take on the role of observer and evaluator of the student in the nurse role. When the assignment is complete the faculty member will engage the students in a debriefing session. Usually the simulation activity is videotaped and used during the debriefing process. During debriefing, the students can discuss how they felt in their roles during the simulation assignment.

Standardized patients can also be used in clinical-based minor assignments. These are either simulated or real patients that have been given a script and coached to role-play the part of a specific patient. As with the high-fidelity simulators, the standardized patient will provide the clinical picture in an identical way to each student, providing consistency in the evaluation process.

Brief Presentation

The brief presentation is different from the presentation discussed as a major assignment because it requires little preparation outside of class and is very specific in focus, such as the written assignments discussed earlier in this chapter. For example, students may be expected to present their work with their assigned patients in a clinical conference.

Brief presentations give students the opportunity to practice expressing and sometimes defending their ideas in an open forum. Give each student guidelines about the objective of the presentation and the detail and areas of emphasis required (e.g., the student may be expected to focus on the admission procedure and related care plan). Students may be required to use a PowerPoint presentation or other computer-based technology for presenting the information. Also, the faculty member should provide the group with guidelines on how to behave in such a forum, the importance of active listening, and ground rules for providing feedback. Students are actively engaged in well-designed brief presentations. Although the individual student does the major work, the remaining students must be attentive if they are to provide meaningful constructive feedback to their colleague. As with other minor assignments, evaluations may be used as a function for giving credit to the student for simply completing it rather than trying to evaluate it in the way one would a major presentation.

Debates

Assign students or ask them to volunteer to argue for or against a proposition. Require them to work in teams or as individuals to develop their arguments. Specify in advance how long the students will have to present their sides as well as the time permitted for rebuttal. Following the debate, the rest of the class can respond to the strength and validity of the arguments. As with other assignments, be explicit about all the parameters involved, such as time, resources used, clarity of presentation, and so on, just as with other presentations.

TOOLS

Designing the Assignment

Start with a concise description of the assignment and the objectives to be met. Describe the expected format and the content to be included. Give the students a sample of what is required in the assignment or guidelines to follow. Minor assignments are always done on an individual basis. These assignments are oriented to individual activities, such as reading or analysis and synthesis of a personal experience.

Grading the Assignment

Minor assignments are frequently given credit just for being completed according to expectations and submitted at the proper time. If you as the faculty member plan to grade a minor assignment, be clear about the criteria and keep them reasonably in accord with the extent of the work required. Specify the requirements for submission or completion. If multiples of a minor assignment are required, such as short essays, specify the intervals at which they are to be submitted.

Minor assignments take little time to grade but may still be time-consuming, especially if multiples are required several times during a term. Students' submitted written work should be evaluated by a method such as a brief written comment. If finding time to evaluate students' work is a problem, then decrease the requirements and expectations. Evaluating students work is an important task, and adequate time must be assigned to read and evaluate student submissions. Designing simulation assignments take a lot of faculty time and effort but have the advantage of observing and evaluating the student in an environment closely mimicking the real clinical situation. Students enjoy these assignments, and anything faculty can do to excite and engage the student in their learning is worth the effort involved. It is common to assign too much work the first time one teaches a course. Talk to colleagues who have taught the same course or similar courses to find out about the amount of work students can handle and how to evaluate their abilities reasonably.

FINAL WORDS

Minor assignments can help evaluate skills difficult to test by objective means. They permit the student to demonstrate specific abilities in a brief format. Although minor, this type of assignment is a valuable resource in the faculty member's toolbox.

FURTHER READING

Issenberg, S. B., Mcgaghie, W. C., Petrusa, E. R., Gordon, D. L., & Scalese, R. J. (2005). Features and uses of high-fidelity medical simulations that lead to effective learning: A BEME systematic review. *Medical Teacher, 27*(1), 10–28. doi:10.1080/01421590500046924

Jeffries, P. R. (2005). A framework for designing, implementing, and evaluating simulations used as teaching strategies in nursing. *Nursing Education Perspectives, 26*(2), 96–103.

Koklanarisa, N., MacKenzieb, A. P., Finoa, M. E., Arslana, A. A., & Seubert, D. E. (2008). Debate preparation/participation: An active, effective learning tool. *Teaching and Learning in Medicine, 20*(3), 235–238. doi:10.1080/10401330802199534

McKeachie, W. J. (2002). *Teaching tips: Strategies, research, and theory for college university teachers* (11th ed.). Boston: Houghton Mifflin.

Vessey, J. A., & Huss, K. (2002). Using standardized patients in advanced practice nursing education. *Journal of Professional Nursing, 18*(1), 29–35. doi:10.1053/jpnu.2002.30898

Test Construction and Analysis

Tests can be used as assessment or evaluation tools and are an inevitable part of teaching. Prior to a class, a test may be used to assess the students' knowledge of a particular topic. The results can be used to help the faculty member plan the course content in a way that meets the needs of the class. After teaching a class, tests are one way to evaluate the students' grasp of the material as well as to assess the faculty member's success at conveying the material. It is important to think of testing in this two-dimensional manner: The better the test, the better evaluation of both the students and faculty. Other methods of evaluation such as case studies, group projects, and papers are increasingly common in classes, but testing remains a high priority, particularly in undergraduate courses, due to the format of the licensing examination. Before planning a test, determine whether it is the most appropriate evaluation tool. Why give a test? If the objectives to be evaluated relate to the lower cognitive levels (i.e., knowledge, comprehension, application), a test may be the most efficient way to find out if the students learned the content of the class. If the objectives pertain to psychomotor skills, the best way to evaluate is to observe the students as they perform the skills. Some students might be able to describe all the steps of a skill in the right order but may not be able to demonstrate the skill correctly or safely. On the other hand, some students may have difficulty in describing the skill, but they can demonstrate it well and safely.

For higher level cognitive objectives or objectives in the affective domain, it is difficult to write test items, especially for an objective test. Other types of assignments, such as those described in Chapters 9 and 10, may often better measure such objectives.

GOALS

The primary goal of testing is to evaluate the ability of students to achieve the desired outcomes as described by course objectives. Testing of students helps to identify gaps in the learning process. The faculty member can assess how the students are learning during the course and adjust the course to help the students achieve the objectives. Another goal of testing is summative evaluation, where the faculty member assesses the student's achievement at the end of the course. Secondarily, testing of students may help in evaluating the effectiveness of the teacher in helping the students to achieve the desired outcomes.

CONTEXT OF TESTING

Before beginning to make use of the tools related to testing, consider the context in which tests are used. Part of planning a course is determining how much testing is needed to assess the students' achievement of course objectives. If the course content is complex and extensive, more tests or alternative assessment strategies may be required. An example would be a course with advanced theory and practical applications, such as a senior year course. In courses in which the content is abstract and where other assignments determine part of the course grade, there will be fewer tests. For example, fewer tests are needed in a course focusing on trends and issues. In such a course, subjective assignments, such as papers or presentations, are more suitable.

Frequency of Tests

Tests should be given at reasonable intervals during a course to allow appropriate time for the students to learn the content. If there are several small tests and a final examination, each small test should cover the same amount of content, have about the same number of items, and be given at regular intervals.

Weighting Tests

The value of each test in determining the course grade should be based on the amount of content each one covers. All tests of a similar nature, such as unit tests, should be given the same weight unless there is a difference in the amount of content covered. Unless tests given early in the course are short or cover less important material, they should be considered equally with later tests. The exception would be for comprehensive examinations, such as a final exam, which would probably be longer and therefore would be given more weight. When considering the weighting of the test, also consider whether the test is given in class and with closed book, or online and with open book. If the test is given online, then the faculty member also needs to consider the length of time the link to the test will be available, whether the test must be completed in one session, or if the student can access the test multiple times during the access period. All of these aspects will factor into the weight of the test. Finally, with an online test, the faculty member needs to have a back-up plan if, for some reason, there are technological difficulties, such as the student being unable to access the test or the Internet connection failing while the student takes the test. An example of the master plan for giving tests in a course is discussed in the following section on test plans.

TOOLS

Test Plans

A test plan is sometimes called a *test blueprint*. As both names suggest, these are tools that help in planning the content for tests.

Course Test Plan

It is important to develop a master plan for all the tests in the course before developing individual test plans. For example, if the course is fairly complex, the faculty member may decide to have three unit tests plus a comprehensive final examination. Table 11.1 shows a course test plan for such a situation. Also, to make sure the faculty member is planning to meet the course objectives, it is beneficial to map the course test plan to the course objectives.

In preparing a course test plan, take into account such things as class periods in which little actual content may be conveyed, such as the first day of class when much time is spent discussing the orientation to the course. Other periods could include spring break or

TABLE 11.1   Course Test Plan

Date	Test	Content	Items	Weight (%)
2/15	Unit 1	Weeks 1–5	60	20
3/21	Unit 2	Weeks 6–10	60	20
4/20	Unit 3	Weeks 11–15	60	20
5/2	Final	Weeks 16 +		
		Comprehensive	120	40

holidays that preempt course time. Finally, it is a good idea to avoid giving a test in the last week of classes in order to help students get ready for final exams. Some schools have policies that require that the last class week be free of tests. Overall, try to come up with a balance so that each test covers the same amount of content, and each content area can is adequately tested. Also, it may be appropriate to evaluate some of the objectives with evaluation strategies such as papers or group assignments. The faculty member must plan to have the due dates for these at different times from the tests along with allowing adequate time for their completion. For the final examination in the example illustrated in Table 11.1, a larger number of items for the content from the last week of class is appropriate, because it had not been previously tested. This portion would include the same number of items as were on the unit tests, as well as additional items that equal the number of items covering each section for the comprehensive part of the final exam.

Individual Test Plan

Although there is a fairly standard way to produce a grid for a test plan, each teacher has to decide what will constitute the parameters. The parameters depend on the type of course and the thrust of the course. For example, a simple plan might have the lectures' content on one axis and the parts of the nursing process on the other. This type of plan is appropriate for many of the nursing courses that are linked to clinical situations such as medical-surgical nursing or pediatrics. Such a plan with equal weightings for each cell is shown in Table 11.2. A more complex plan may have the lecture content on one axis and the taxonomy of cognitive objectives on the other. This plan is particularly useful in courses such as pharmacology or genetics.

The sample test plan in Table 11.2 shows the lecture numbers on the vertical axis. For clarity, an abbreviated version of the lecture title, such

TABLE 11.2   Test Plan Without Differential Weightings for Cells

	Assess	Plan	Implement	Evaluate	Total
Lec. 1	3	3	3	3	12
Lec. 2	3	3	3	3	12
Lec. 3	3	3	3	3	12
Lec. 4	3	3	3	3	12
Totals	12	12	12	12	48

as "Immobility" or "ADL" could be listed in each space. The horizontal axis indicates the parts of the nursing process with a final column heading for row totals.

The grid in Table 11.2 was constructed by simply multiplying the number of columns by the number of rows. This gave the number of cells (16). Presume that there was 60 minutes available for the testing period. The students were given about 1 minute per item; the time available was divided by the number of cells (60 ÷ 16 = 3.75). In Table 11.2, each cell has a 3 in it. Next, it was decided to have the same number of items for each cell, and the number had to be a round number, thus the result rounded (3.75) up to 4 and then multiplied by the number of cells to get the total items for the test (4 x 16 = 64). Therefore 64 items were required, which would be pushing some students to respond in 60 minutes. However, with the number rounded down to 3, which resulted in a requirement of a total of 48 items. Table 11.3 summarizes these steps.

The plan in Table 11.2 was based on the assumption that the content to be tested in each cell was equally important as the content in every other cell. As a matter of fact, it is possible and perhaps important to put greater weight on some aspects than on others. The sample plan shown in Table 11.4 reflects a situation in which judgments have been made about the differential weighting of content.

In developing the sample plan in Table 11.4, the first step is to determine the number of items in each cell of the plan. To do this, decide on priorities about the most important content covered by the plan. The first question to ask is, "How should each component of the horizontal axis be weighted?" In the sample plan, the implementation step of the nursing process should be weighted more heavily than the other steps. About a third of the resultant test would be on that step. The assessment and planning phases are weighted equally with one another. The evaluation step would have fewer items, because the class was an early

TABLE 11.3 Calculating Number of Items per Cell When Weightings Are Equal

Step 1: Rows x columns = number of cells

Step 2: Time for test ÷ number of cells = items per cell

Step 3: If items per cell is not a round number, round it up or down so that items per cell x number of cells ≤ time for test

TABLE 11.4 Test Plan Based on Lecture Content and Parts of the Nursing Process With Differential Weighting of Content[a]

	Assess	Plan	Implement	Evaluate	Total
Lec. 1	**2.75/3**	**2.75/3**	**3.67/4**	**1.83/2**	**11/12**
Lec. 2	**2.75/2**	**2.75/2**	**3.67/4**	**1.83/2**	**11/10**
Lec. 3	**2.75/3**	**2.75/2**	**3.67/4**	**1.83/2**	**11/11**
Lec. 4	**2.75/2**	**2.75/3**	**3.67/4**	**1.83/2**	**11/11**
Lec. 5	2/2	2/2	**3.67/3**	**1.33/0**	8/7
Lec. 6	2/3	2/2	**2.67/3**	**1.33/1**	8/9
Totals	**15/15**	**15/14**	**20/22**	**10/9**	**60/60**

[a]The projected number of items for each cell is shown in bold. The number on the right side of the slash in each cell represents the actual number planned for the test.

course in which students might be expected to have little skill in the evaluation aspect.

The next question is, "How should the content on the vertical axis be weighted?" In the sample in Table 11.4, the content in the first four lectures was of equal importance. However, the last two lectures were not given as much weight. A situation like this would be one in which the first four lectures cover complex content, which might require more items to sample the students' knowledge adequately. The last lectures might be as long, but they would include less complex content or content that could be tested more easily with fewer questions.

The test being planned in Table 11.4 would be given in a 60-minute period, so that gave the grand total for the number of items. The decisions about the axes led to the assignment of hypothetical totals for each row and column. To calculate the number of items that would fit into each cell, the column and row totals for that cell were multiplied, and then divided by the total number of items. For example, for the cell under "Assessment" for the first lecture, 15 multiplied by 11 and divided by 60 equals 2.75.

In order to arrive at the actual numbers for each cell in Table 11.4, round the fractional numbers up or down. To determine which direction to go, consider what content was being tested within each cell. For each lecture, look at each lecture objective and see what was emphasized. For the first lecture, the first three steps in the nursing process were about equally emphasized in the objectives and content, and should have the maximum number of items to sample the students' knowledge. However, it may be that those two items would be sufficient to indicate if a student could adequately evaluate the success of the earlier steps in dealing with the topic.

For every decision to round a projected number up or down, a number in another cell had to be rounded in the opposite direction so that the final total of items would be correct. In the hypothetical test in Table 11.4, it was decided that two items were sufficient for testing both assessment and planning for the second lecture. These numbers were then rounded down to accommodate numbers that were increased. In one column where all the numbers were rounded up, the new total was higher than the projected total. Because this column was to be weighted heavily, then lower totals were accepted in two other columns.

Another factor to note is that one cell is empty. Sometimes the content may not lend itself to any items in a given cell, or it might be expected that the students will not be able to answer items about it because there is not a relevant lecture objective pertaining to that knowledge. This example shows that even though there is a technical way to calculate the item totals, professional judgment should be used to determine the final number of items for each cell. Remember, it is not necessary to test every cell in the grid.

Some situations call for only one item, whereas others require more than one to test an objective. An objective on the cognitive level of knowledge could be "Define cardiomyopathy." One item could sufficiently determine if students could do this. Higher level objectives would not only require more complex items, but also more items. For example, "Develop an evaluation plan for the care of a patient with heart failure" might require several objective items or one short answer item worth several points.

Although in the example the values in the cells of the test plan have been referred to as equivalent to numbers of items, one could think of these as numbers of points. For example, in the evaluation cell for Lecture No. 1, there could be two multiple-choice items worth one point each, or one short-answer item worth two points.

Test-Item Bank

The faculty member should develop a system to store items electronically for future tests. There are many software programs available for this purpose. These programs allow categorization and filing of items with a variety of descriptors so that a set of test items that meet certain criteria can be reviewed. For example, all the items on specific nursing interventions for a heart failure patient can be selected. Then, from the items available, the number required for the test plan can be selected. These programs also allow the computer to select the number of items required from those stored.

It is standard in most nursing textbooks to include a test-item bank such as Examview, which is available in a downloadable format or with instructor texts on computer disks. These items may be based directly on the content in the respective texts, of course, but it is usually possible to edit the items as well as to add new items to the bank. Other texts have a companion instructor manual that contains test items for the purpose of supplementing your personal bank. These are good sources because the items are already categorized and referenced to the text. Although the instructor may still wish to produce test items, these sources can help to give more variety and provide many questions each content area. Some publishers provide online instructor's guides for the textbooks that include test items related to each chapter. It is crucial that the faculty member review the published test items before using them to ensure that the items will indeed test that the students are achieving the course objectives.

Proficiency Examinations

Many schools have provisions for students to challenge courses. This means the student may earn credit other than by enrolling in a course. One way this may be done is by a teacher-made proficiency examination. A proficiency exam should be based on the same fundamental elements as the course. Examinees should be required to show that they know at least as much as the average student who took the course and passed it.

If part of the course grade is determined by means other than tests, the process to challenge should include the same means. For example, if the course has a practical component such as doing a physical assessment or demonstrating other psychomotor skills, a portion of the exam should replicate that aspect. In a beginning research course, students may have to pass written exams and critique a research report. The same performance would be expected of those who challenge the course.

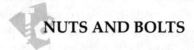

NUTS AND BOLTS

Types of Items

Objective

The most common items are objective items. The objectivity involved means that the correct answer is objectively determined. The students must choose from answers provided. Examples of these types of items are multiple choice, multiple response, true/false, and matching. Most students have probably been exposed to all of these, but each kind will be described briefly here.

Multiple-choice items include a stem that describes a person or situation and asks a question about it. The student must select the correct answer from a set of options. A variation on the multiple-choice item is the multiple-response question. However, as opposed to one correct answer in the multiple-choice format, the student must select all answers that apply to the question asked. This means that multiple-response questions are considerably more complicated to answer and write.

True/false items are usually one-sentence statements. The student must decide whether the statement is true or false. Matching items include two lists of terms. The student is asked to match terms from one list with terms on the other list, according to some specification.

Objective items are easy to grade because a test key permits rapid marking or because they can be graded electronically and the item results analyzed. The item-analysis report provides information related to determining the degree of difficulty and the discrimination index for each item that the faculty member can use for future refinement of the items.

Subjective

The subjectivity involved in subjective items is that of the person grading the items. The student is given some latitude in answering, and the teacher determines if the answer is correct. The student must provide an answer without any cues. The basic types are short-answer items, unfolding case studies, and essay questions.

In short-answer items, the student must recall the correct information without the prompting of options. This type of item can either have a question or a fill-in-the-blank format. The question format items calls for a few words or at most a sentence or two to answer the question. The fill-in-the-blank may just need a number or word for the answer. Short-answer items are close to objective items because there is usually only one correct response. Unfolding case studies are a useful method to test critical-thinking skills because they mirror situations in clinical practice. The faculty member develops a case study similar to situations in the clinical arena with changes in the patient's condition. Following the introduction of the case, there are questions for the student. Then, as the case study unfolds and new information about the patient's condition or setting is given, there are questions at each stage of the unfolding of the case. The construction of this type of test question relies heavily on up-to-date clinical experience. An essay question requires a lengthy response and calls for the student to demonstrate more than simply recalling facts. The student may be expected to demonstrate high-level cognitive objectives, such as analysis or synthesis. Essay items may be used to test students' ability to meet objectives in the affective domain.

Subjective items take longer to grade. With short-answer items, it takes a little longer to recognize a word or phrase as the answer sheet is scanned than to simply recognize if the correct letter of the right option has been filled in. With lengthy answers, even more time is required to read and evaluate the students' responses. The faculty member may decide to restrict the essay response to a paragraph or two. With this instruction, the student has to discern the most salient information rather than including everything they know on the topic. The advantage for the faculty member is that grading takes less time and students receive their results more quickly.

Writing Test Items

A good test item should meet the following criteria: (1) It relates to important content that the students should retain; (2) it is unambiguous; and (3) if it is an objective item, it has one and only one correct answer among the choices provided. In addition to these criteria, there are several other important principles to consider in writing items.

The majority of the following principles pertain to objective items, but some would pertain to either type of item as well as specifically for subjective items

1. *Significance of content.* If you ask the students to respond to an item on a test, it should be important for them to know the specific piece of information they are being asked about. It would be easy to ask for something specific, such as, "When are immunizations for pertussis, rubella, polio, and tetanus given in the first year of a child's life?" The options could be a laundry list of time intervals. Is this information they should memorize? How long will they retain it if they do? It might be more valuable to ask a question such as, "What would be the most effective way to help a mother of a small child to remember when to get her child's immunizations?" This is a higher level question, and it also tests for application that would be transferable to other nursing situations. Faculty must teach the content and test it at the same level; for example, content must not be taught in the cognitive level or at the knowledge level but tested at the analysis level. The faculty member must make sure there is consistency; otherwise, the students will not succeed on their tests. Frequently in baccalaureate programs, faculty members test the more complex content that is common in the program and may never ask simple questions on basic nursing practice. Baccalaureate graduates may be able to answer questions on metabolism at the cellular level, and yet not be able to recognize a diet high in vitamin C. The critical question is, "What will the graduates need to know to be safe, competent, beginning practitioners at their level of preparation?"

2. *Clarity.* The item should be easy to read, so that the students spend their time thinking about the correct answer rather than trying to decipher the meaning of the question. Use vocabulary that is common to what the students read for the course. Use simple terms they are likely to know, unless recognizing the terminology is part of what you are testing. Do not use abbreviation of terms unless the term is spelled out initially followed by the abbreviation in parentheses.

Make sure that your stem and your options are as unambiguous as possible. An example of an ambiguous stem would be, "Mr. Warren is receiving Prozac. One morning he asks his nurse the name of the drug. She tells him it is to help his mood. What is this called?" Once the student reads the options, the stem may seem less ambiguous, but initially, it is probably not clear what the word *this* refers to. Does it mean the reason for the patient's question, or does it refer to the nurse's response? A less ambiguous question would be, "What would the nurse's response be called?"

3. *One correct answer.* The correct answer may not be comprehensive, but it should be correct and should answer the question in the stem. For example, in response to the question, "Which of the following is a reason people experience crisis?" a correct answer would be, "Lack of a support system." There are other correct answers that contribute, but this is a correct answer even by itself. None of the other options should be true. If there could be several correct answers but one is more important or more significant, the others can be used as distracters, but the stem must make clear that the students are to choose the most significant answer from the options

4. *Clear basis for a correct response.* The criterion for what the student must choose as the correct response should be clearly indicated. For example, what would be the correct response to the following sample item?

Mr. Carson complains at length about his pains in his feet and back. No pathology has been discovered to account for this pain, and the staff believes this complaining is a symptom of low self-esteem and need for attention. When Mr. Carson begins complaining to you, what would you say?

a. "You are just seeking attention."
b. "I will sit and talk with you for awhile."
c. "If you quit talking about the pain, it will go away."
d. "I will come back when you feel better."

Even though option "b" is the most therapeutic choice, because the stem asked the student "What would you say?" any answer could be correct. Specify the criterion by which the right answer is to be determined (e.g., use such phrases as the *best thing to say (or do); the first thing; the highest priority; the most helpful*). The person who is taking action should be the nurse, or the student assuming the role of the nurse. Then ask, "What should the nurse say?"

5. *Believable distracters.* Each incorrect option should be somewhat believable, so that at least a few students would choose each one.

Distracters must be carefully thought out because they are used to distract the unsure student rather than being used as an obviously incorrect response. Good distracters are things that the average person might think or things that are common misconceptions. The following item helps to illustrate this.

What is the first priority in dealing with a psychotic patient?

a. Decrease the patient's hallucinations
b. Promote the patient's developing trust
c. Improve the patient's self-esteem
d. Increase the patient's interactions with others

An intelligent person who has not been studying psychiatric nursing lately would be likely to think that the most important thing in working with someone who is psychotic is to deal with the most obvious evidence of psychosis, hallucinations. Others might guess such people should interact with other people to help them become less withdrawn. Others who did not really understand working with such patients might think you should focus on low self-esteem, which they recall as part of the psychotic person's problems. The student who understands the fundamental aspects of working with these patients will know that trust is essential to accomplish any of the other goals.

6. *Length.* Each multiple-choice item should take about 1 minute to read and answer. If you want to provide a hypothetical patient to whom the students will refer, include only the data that will apply to the items. The exception to this would be when it is important for the students to demonstrate that they can discriminate between extraneous and important data. Look at the following item and see how much one could delete and still have a good item.

Mary Jones is a 23-year-old married woman with a high school education. She works as a secretary for an oil company. She has been diagnosed as having rheumatoid arthritis. Which of the following would be the most appropriate set of instructions for maintaining her joint mobility?

a. Take aspirin only once a day, and apply heat to joints
b. Exercise moderately, and protect joints from exposure to cold air
c. Eat plenty of green vegetables, and take extra iron
d. Maintain internal rotation of joints, and drink extra fluids

Unless you are planning to have several items pertaining to Mary Jones, the majority of the information in the stem is irrelevant because selecting the correct answer is not dependent upon any of the information specific to the patient. The stem can be cut down to, "In order to maintain joint mobility in a person with rheumatoid arthritis, which of the following would be the most appropriate set of instructions?"

7. *Simple multiple choice.* The current preference among many nursing educators is for simple multiple-choice items rather than multiple-multiple-choice items. A simple multiple-choice item allows specific evaluation of the student's knowledge in that content area. In a multiple-multiple-choice item, a student may choose the correct option by eliminating one of the suboptions, without understanding the reason for the correct answer. Another benefit of simple multiple-choice items is that these prepare the students for the RN licensing examination.

8. *Distribution of correct answers.* Keep track of the letters or numbers of the correct options for items written. Over the test as a whole, each option should be the correct answer about the same number of times. Keep a tally as items are written for a test. If using some previously written items, note the correct options to start with so that the equal numbers can be maintained. This helps to prevent students from answering correctly just because they may have noticed a tendency to have the third option as the correct one a lot of the time. To avoid this problem completely, alphabetize the options in descending order. If the subsequent option begins with the same word, go to the next word to sort in alphabetical order

9. *Options with numbers.* When using options with numbers, each option should be exclusive. For example:

What is the acceptable dosage of diazepam (Valium) for treatment of anxiety?

a. 2 mg b.i.d.
b. 4–40 mg daily
c. 20–40 mg daily
d. Up to 50 mg

Yikes! Where is the student to start in sorting this one out? The second option is correct in terms of being the range of acceptable doses, but 20 to 40 mg is included within that range. The first option is correct as a daily dose even though it does not reflect a range. The fourth option is the only one that is clearly unacceptable.

Numbers should make sense for the situation being described. Values that are too small or too large are unlikely to be chosen. They should also be in the same type of measurement, such as all in milligrams or all in ounces, unless part of what the item is testing is the ability of the student to convert from one system of measurement to another. It is usually best to present numbers in increments from small to large.

10. *Cues to the right answer.* Be careful to avoid echoing words from the stem in the correct option. The following example shows this error.

    What process do nurses use in caring for patients?

    a. Problem solving
    b. Scientific approach
    c. Nursing process
    d. Analysis

Another inadvertent clue would be to use a plural reference in the stem when only the correct option contains a plural noun.

    Which people are at highest risk for committing suicide?

    a. Teenagers
    b. A professional
    c. An old person
    d. A woman

Avoid direct quotes in options unless all of the options sound the same.

    What is the definition of "ethnocentrism"?

    a. Thinking your culture is the center of the universe
    b. Having a God-oriented belief system
    c. The belief that one's own cultural or social group is superior to others
    d. Failing to take culture into account in working with patients

The third option sounds like a textbook definition of a term whereas the incorrect options begin with a gerund and do not sound as formal. This could be corrected by restating the other options in parallel language, such as the statements below:

> The idea that one's culture is the center of the universe
>
> The presence of a belief system that is God-oriented
>
> The tendency to exclude cultural concerns from interactions

11. *"None of the above" and "All of the above."* If you use options like "None of the above" or "All of the above," there are some things to keep in mind.

    Sometimes include these options when they are wrong as well as when they are correct.

    When including "None of the above," indicate in the stem that the student may expect this option. For example, "Which of the following, if any, would be the right breathing technique for a woman in the first stage of labor?"

    Do not overuse "All of the above" just because it may be difficult to come up with three good distracters for each item. This makes the test much easier than if the students had to make real discriminations.

12. *Using negatives.* Stems that ask students questions couched in negative terms are more difficult to read and may inadvertently trick the students. If using a negative term or if asking for the reverse of what is usually asked, emphasize it in some way to draw the students' attention. Some examples are, "Which of the following would not be an appropriate toy for a 4-year-old child in the hospital?" or "What would be the least effective treatment for a strained muscle?" Be careful about introducing double negatives, which may confound the students' understanding. For example:

    Stem: When would you not suggest a patient cough and deep breathe after surgery?

    Option: When he or she is not receiving artificial ventilation.

13. *Stereotyped or sexist language.* Take as much care to respect the rights and feelings of students when writing test items as when interacting with them in person. The following are some problems encountered by nursing faculty when writing test items.

Attributing unintelligent or negative qualities to hypothetical patients or nurses who are in particular ethnic or gender groups: "Maria Gomez is a poorly educated woman with a history of child abuse." It is appropriate that some items on your test should have different ethnic groups represented, but be sure that they are not included only in negative contexts.

- Attaching names that have been used with unflattering connotations for certain ethnic groups: "Jemimah is a black woman who does not understand conception control."
- Implying that one gender is not as bright or as good as the other: "Paul is a straight A student, while Mary is barely passing."
- Implying that patients of one gender are only interested in stereotyped activities or involved in certain roles. An example of this would be leaving the father out when discussing hypothetical situations relating to children.
- Neglecting to use male names for any of the hypothetical nurses in your test items or making all the nurses women and most of the patients men (unless you are dealing with obstetrics).
- Using certain ethnic groups' names when describing aggressive or other behaviors that may have negative connotations.

To avoid these pitfalls, do not make everyone a Smith, Jones, or Garcia. Try to use typical sounding names from a variety that have different ethnic origins. If comparing two people, one of who has a negative attribution, make both the people of the same gender and same ethnic group. However, it is best to avoid using names altogether and to use neutral terms such as patient, client, or nurse. This way no one will be offended by the test items.

14. *Bias in tests.* There is a relationship between English proficiency and examination performance. In developing tests, make certain that your exams do not include terms and expressions that students with English as a second language (ESL) may not know. Test items may be culturally biased if culturally specific knowledge is needed to answer the question correctly. Students not of part of this cultural group will statistically provide incorrect responses to the question more often that those students from the cultural group. To reduce this cultural bias the faculty member must include the cultural aspects related to the specific patient condition

in the class content. An example of this is the ethic and cultural aspects of sickle cell disease. However, regardless of the cultural makeup of the student class, the faculty member must include in a test questions of this condition and its related cultural components because it is a common condition seen in clinical practice.

15. *Introduce humor with care.* Some faculty members like to include one or two items intended to be funny for the purpose of relieving tension. Ironically, this maneuver sometimes has the opposite effect. If the attempt is ambiguous or if the students are so engrossed in the testing process that they overlook the intent, they may become distracted. If an item is meant to be funny, either make it the last one or tag it clearly as such. Once again, the use of humor in testing with a diverse student body may introduce a cultural bias. Many ESL students may not understand or appreciate the humor and in fact may become more confused.

16. *Specify response length.* When writing short-answer or essay questions, indicate how much of a response is expected. For example, with a short answer item, provide a blank to fill in that limits the length of the response. Make sure the blank is of sufficient length to accommodate the expected response. An example would be: "What is the average age at which infants' teeth first emerge? ____months"

For essay questions, specify not only the length, but make any other applicable parameters clear. The following two examples show this.

> Example 1: Using 100 to 125 words, identify and discuss one of the major contributions Florence Nightingale made to the foundation of modern nursing. Describe the impact of her innovation on nursing as it was practiced in her era.

> Example 2: Select a situation with ethical implications from the following: abortion, total life support, sterilization, death and dying, in vitro fertilization. State your position and analyze how you arrived at your position using either a deontological or a teleological model. Your response should be around 250 words.

Assembling a Test

There are some technical aspects to putting the test together that will make it look polished and ensure that the students will not be at a disadvantage because of extraneous factors that have nothing to do with their knowledge.

Order

Make sure you allow plenty of time to assemble the test and put it in the final format. When assembling a test, one idea is to put the items in the same order as the content was presented in class. This means that all items over one part of the content are together. It also means that they are most likely in order from less difficult to more difficult within each group. Another idea is to put all the questions with the same format together, for example, all the multiple choice. With this method, the student stays in the groove or mindset for that type of response before moving on to perhaps short-answer questions. Another option available with computerized test administration is presenting the questions in random order. This has advantages if the students are doing this test outside class because they cannot just give each other the list of responses they think match the questions.

Arrangement

The beginning and ending of the components of each item should be clear. All the parts of an item should be on the same page. For example, do not have the stem on one page and the options or part of the options on another. All items should be presented in a standard format. The examples given earlier in this chapter show a standard format.

Clear directions for the student are essential. The time allowed should be clearly written at the beginning of the test. Explain clearly what you want the student to do for each question or group of questions. If it is a computerized test, make sure the student knows whether they can go back to a previous question to change an answer before they submit the test. On the last page of the test, provide clear instructions about how to hand in or submit the test electronically.

Options

In a multiple-choice item, the options should always be listed in the same way (e.g., in a vertical list). List every set of options either flush with the left margin or aligned along an indent of the same number of spaces each time.

Each item should have the same number of options, preferably four. It is difficult to come up with four distracters for each item, as is needed with five options for each item. Three options are too few because it increases the possibility of students' getting the correct answer by chance. Another reason to use the same number of options for each item is to avoid causing the student to make a mistake, such as marking "d" when they mean to choose the last option, which might be "e."

Proofing

Always proofread your own tests. Having another faculty member read it may help to identify errors also. Make sure each item is complete and that they are all arranged in the chosen format. Check for misspellings or missing words. Be especially alert for negative words that may have been omitted.

Administration of Tests

The faculty member must decide whether the test will be administered face to face or online, and if it will be a pencil-and-paper or computer-based test. Students must be informed early in the course about these expectations. Check with the students about their computer and Internet access. If they lack these resources, it will make the decision to have the test in class and face to face easy.

The advent of hybrid (mixed format of in class and online) or online courses often necessitates the use of an open-book test. This type of testing allows students to use their books and notes as resources for an examination. Students may believe that this type of test is easier than a traditional exam, but on examination, open-book tests have been found to be equally difficult to traditional testing. The faculty member who chooses to use open-book testing must assist students in understanding the different preparation requirements for both the traditional examinations and open-book examinations. Students may think that they do not have to study and know the material if they can access their books and course notes during the test. They may spend so much time searching for the answers they do not have sufficient time to complete the test.

Cheating is a growing concern for faculty, particularly with all the technology available. On the first day of class, a review of the academic integrity policy along with posting a copy on the course-management site for the students will increase awareness of this issue. Prior to a test, some faculty members may ask students to turn off all technology-related items, including cell phones, while others may collect all of these items and return them once the test is completed. Ensure there are sufficient faculty and teaching assistants present to proctor the test. For online tests, students use their ID and password to access the test site. Usually the test is held on the course-management system and is secure. Limit the time for the test to the same length it would be if it were given in class. Allow the student to access the test site once. Provide the student with guidelines about next steps if the student gets locked out of the site while taking the test. There are a number of reasons this may occur, ranging from a break in the Internet service to the student trying to print the test. The faculty member may have a rule that students who have got locked out of the site must come to the school, meet with the faculty member within a short time span, and take the test there.

Grading Tests

There is no need to hand-grade multiple-choice items. If grading tests by hand, do everything possible in advance to simplify the procedure. This would include having answer sheets separate from the test itself. Set them up so that the scoring key can easily be aligned with the answers for ease in reading and marking. If giving subjective tests that have to be hand-graded, plan ahead of time to allow for the time needed to grade the papers. Prepare a grading rubric for each of these questions to reduce subjectivity. Often, teaching assistants can be valuable in assisting with grading subjective tests

Test Analysis

Most educational institutions have centralized computer services to calculate test reliability and item analysis. The usual data provided are an alphabetical listing of the students with their individual raw score, percentage score, and percentage rank. Also included is the number of students, number of items on the test, maximum possible score, mean score, mean percentage score, standard deviation, and a frequency distribution of scores. For teacher-made tests, reliabilities between 0.60 and 0.80 are considered good, if there are about 50 to 60 questions and more than, say, 15 students—and no keying errors. The reliability of a

test can be increased by making it longer. Even though it seems difficult to write more items on an area of content, there are many possible
items that could be asked about any subject. If asking a dozen questions about proper ways to position an immobilized patient, a student
who really understands the principles should be able to get most of
the questions right. However, even a good student could miss 2 of 12
items on the subject. What if only two questions were asked, and those
two questions were the ones the student did not know? On the other
hand, a weak student might answer only half the items on positioning,
but one of the six could be one of the two the other student answered
incorrectly. This would give a different picture of the students' knowledge. Therefore, the more items, the better the indication you get of
the strengths and weaknesses of your students. If it is possible to add
some items, especially on a complex area of content, even a little may
help to make your results more reliable.

Item Analysis

Item analysis is used to help determine the content validity of the test.
Did the test measure what it was supposed to measure?

Information provided by an item analysis helps to improve items
before they are used again. It also quickly reveals if there were clearly
no correct answer or if the wrong answer were keyed as correct. The
item analysis will tell the number of students who responded to each
option. It will also indicate the difficulty of the item. Depending on
how the data are presented, an easy question is determined on the
basis that nearly everyone answered it correctly. When there are questions that a high number of students have missed, examine them to
be sure they are fair. Maybe a lot of students missed them because
they were not well written, or the material may not have been covered
well enough for them to have understood the important points. On
the other hand, when the correlation between a given item and the
whole test is examined, it may be concluded that the item is a good
discriminator between the better and the weaker students. This will be
discussed further later on.

Evaluating Distractors

By looking at the percentages of students who chose incorrect options, one
can more easily evaluate how well the distractors are working. If no

one ever selects a certain distractor after an item is used two or three times, there is no point in having it there. Try a new distractor or try rewriting it to make the item more challenging. If one distractor gets chosen about as often as the correct option, this may give an indication of areas of content that are difficult for students to understand. This information is beneficial when planning the content and teaching methods for the next class.

Discrimination

Sometimes the correlation value between the item and the test is referred to as the discrimination power because it shows how well the item helps to discriminate between the students who do well on the test and those who do not.

The discrimination power is a helpful statistic. A statistically significant value indicates that the particular item is doing a good job of differentiating among the students' performances on the test. These items help to identify who should be in the various groups for grades. However, if too many of the items have high discrimination power, the test may be too difficult for the group you are testing.

Because this is a correlation statistic, the values range from −1.0 to +1.0. Items with values around 0 to 0.30 are usually not discriminating. Items with negative values are negatively correlated with the test as a whole. This is fairly unusual, especially to see a negative correlation that is significant. This result means that students who do well on the test are tending to miss the item. This could be because there is some room for interpretation and the better students read more into the question or understand the information better.

Revising Items

The data from the statistics will help with improving the items. Some of the ways in which this helps have already been mentioned. When first reviewing the statistics, make notes about obvious problems. However, it is often better to allow some time before working on revisions, because it may result in rewriting better test items. Time will give you objectivity when evaluating these items.

Have other faculty members review the items. Even if the content is not their area of expertise, they can identify process strengths and weaknesses in the items. Because they do not necessarily know the content, they can sometimes pick out ways in which the correct answer is cued by the stem. They can recognize ambiguous items because they do not know the content to the degree the item writers do. Do not be reluctant to strike a deal with a colleague on the faculty in a different specialty to exchange items for evaluation.

Obviously, it is also helpful to ask colleagues with the same specialty to read the items. They can validate the content as well as give ideas about what is significant enough to test. Listen to the advice that is given and use it to improve items that need improvement.

Validity of Proficiency Exams

In order to tell if a proficiency test is doing what it is supposed to do, compare the test performance of people who have not taken the course to those who have. If the same exam is used in both groups, simply look at the performance of students who enrolled in the course compared to the challengers. However, if a different exam is used for the proficiency exam, bias could be introduced that makes the test too hard or too easy compared to what is required of those who enroll.

Student Review of Tests

Students should get feedback on their test grades within a week or so after they take the test. One hotly contested issue about tests is how to give the students feedback about their performance and whether or not to give tests back to students to keep. One reason given for not letting students see their exams is to protect the test-item bank; however, if the test-item bank is big enough, it does not matter.

If students are able to see their tests without keeping them, schedule a time for students to review the test. Focus on answering questions about rationale, and make the review a learning experience. If the students have complaints, let them put their concerns in writing. Provide opportunity to review items that were particularly difficult for students to grasp, discussing the rationale behind the correct answer.

Student feedback can also be provided by having a copy of the exam with the correct answers marked available for them to view at designated times and for a limited time period after the exam. If this method of feedback is used, set some ground rules, such as that the merits of the exam or individual items will not be discussed.

In some schools, tests are routinely given back to students to assist them in their own review. Files of old tests are maintained and are available to all students, not just those with friends in the previous class.

Student Reactions

Feelings always run high about tests. It is tough for students to always be subjected to being tested. Because tests frequently constitute a major portion of a course grade, students are concerned about the impact of each test and of each item on their final grades. They can and will argue long and hard for one or two more points. Many teachers are surprised and perplexed about the behavior of students in response to tests. Teachers can learn a great deal from the feedback of their students about the fairness and appropriateness of the exam.

A faculty member with a good understanding of all the components of test construction and analysis will be able to provide responses to the students supported by evidence based on the testing. These responses should be tempered with support for the students, and the faculty member must make sure the students understand they that have been heard and that their feedback is an important part of the testing and evaluation process.

FINAL WORDS

Testing helps to assess student learning as well as to evaluate teacher success. The procedures in developing items, assembling exams, and analyzing results are complex, but logical. Producing fair tests is a fundamental skill for nursing faculty, but developing that skill takes time and effort.

OTHER RESOURCES YOU WOULD BE WISE TO CONSIDER

Test-Construction Workshops

Everyone who writes tests ought to go to one test-construction workshop. These workshops provide a good foundation for constructing tests.

Teaching Centers/Test Review Committees

Many educational institutions have teaching centers, and one of the services provided is assistance in test construction. A staff member can provide a workshop on test construction and evaluation for faculty groups.

Some schools have a test review committee. This committee works with new faculty to enhance their test construction skills and provides guidance and support to all faculty members for test-construction issues.

Colleagues

Working with colleagues is an excellent way to improve test-construction skills. Look at their tests and ask them about their judgments. Then ask them to evaluate your items.

Coursework

A formal college course can help faculty to write better tests and understand more about the statistics involved. If you are planning to enroll in such a course, make sure that the content will address your needs. For example, a course called Tests and Measurements may be described in the college catalog as dealing with test construction, but the bulk of the course may be on statistics.

Educational Testing Service

The Educational Testing Service (ETS) is the leading authority in test development. Many standardized tests used in every level of education and in many professions are developed, printed, or graded by ETS. They provide consultation to groups who are developing major examinations, such as the American Nurses Association Certification Program. They publish many useful monographs about test construction.

FURTHER READING

Aamodt, M. G., & Teige McShane, T. (1992). Meta-analytic investigation of the effect of various test item characteristics on test scores and test completion times. *Public Personnel Management, 21*(2), 151–160.

Bosher, S. (2003). Barriers to creating a more culturally diverse nursing profession: Linguistic bias in multiple-choice nursing exams. *Nursing Education Perspectives, 24*(1), 25–34.

Clifton, S. L., & Schriner, C. L. (2010). Assessing the quality of multiple-choice test items. *Nurse Educator, 35*(1),12–16. doi: 10.1097/NNE.0b 013e3181c41fa3

McDonald, M. (2002). *Systematic assessment of learning outcomes: Developing multiple choice exams.* Sudbury, MA: Jones & Bartlett.

McGahee, T. W., & Ball, J. (2009). How to read and really use an item analysis. *Nurse Educator, 34*(4), 166–171. doi: 10.1097/NNE.0b 013e3181aaba94

McKeachie, W. J. (2002). *Teaching tips: Strategies, research, and theory for college university teachers* (11th ed.). Boston: Houghton Mifflin.

Oermann, M. H., & Gaberson, K. B. (2009). *Evaluation and testing in nursing education* (3rd ed.) New York: Springer.

Oermann, M. H., Saewert, K. J., Charisika, M., & Yarborough, S. S. (2009). Clinical evaluation and grading practices in schools of nursing: National survey findings part I. *Nursing Education Perspectives, 30*(5), 274–279.

Rakes. G. C. (2008). Open book testing in online learning environments. *Journal of Interactive Online Learning, 7*(1), 1541–4914.

Vessey, J. A., & Huss, K. (2002). Using standardized patients in advanced practice nursing education. *Journal of Professional Nursing, 18*(1), 29–35. doi:10.1053/jpnu.2002.30898

Zary, N., Johnson, G., Boberg, J., & Fors, U. G. H. (2006). Development, implementation and pilot evaluation of a Web-based virtual patient case simulation environment—Web-SP. *BMC Medical Education, 6*(10). doi:10.1186/1472–6920–6-10

12

Using Technology to Facilitate Learning

Technology encompasses all educational activities that require and involve the use of a computer. The computer is an essential tool for present-day education, especially with millennial students. Computers are invaluable for writing papers, collecting and storing class notes, preparing projects and presentations, and for communication with classmates, faculty, and the world. For online or distance learning courses, the computer may even be the primary source for access to course materials and instruction. Some other computer-based technological tools to facilitate learning and foster student interactivity are student response systems, lecture capture, high-fidelity simulators, second-life or created virtual-learning environments, asynchronous learning management (LMS) system, synchronous web conferencing software, personal digital assistants (PDAs), and podcasting of educational content. Computerized patient-information systems may also be encountered in hospitals, clinics, and other community institutions used for student clinical experiences. Faculty must be prepared to use a wide variety of technology to meet the students' learning needs as well as address the way students use technology continuously in their everyday interactions. Students multitask with different computer-based applications, and use these computer-based modalities to stay virtually connected rather than being physically present. Faculty needs to provide learning experiences through multiple technological platforms that allow the students to be virtually connected to the course faculty and the rest of the class if the faculty member is to successfully teach the student in this digital age. Faculty must recognize that some students may need a basic computer-literacy course if they do not have minimal computer-literacy skills.

GOALS

The computer's principal use is as a tool to assist students to access, organize, store, retrieve, interact with course content, and communicate information. It may also free faculty from repetitious aspects of teaching and enable faculty to become more of a facilitator of learning and communication.

TOOLS

Hardware

Computer

The type of computer that is used is not as important as access to one. Today, having a computer is as vital to learning as a pen or pencil was in the past. The majority of students will have their own computers, and in many cases this will be a laptop computer. In addition, nursing schools usually have computer labs or media centers that are available for student use. Because many students use the labs, finding a free machine may be a problem. It is important to inform incoming students of the type and minimum computer specifications needed for participating in course and school activities. This is essential for students as many of the courses will involve some aspect of the school's online course-management system. Many academic institutions have financial arrangements for students to purchase computers at a discount rate and/or to take out a financial loan.

Other hardware may be needed in addition and is dependent upon the technology used. Besides a computer, a PDA, a smart phone, or a response key pad (clicker) may be required to access or interact within the course. For example, students who use student-response pads need to purchase and then register the pads online so their responses to questions during a PowerPoint presentation can be tabulated and displayed. Clicker technology is discussed later in this chapter.

Lecture Capture

Lecture capture is another Web-based tool that record PowerPoint lectures along with audio. Students are given access to a Web site where these lectures are stored. Then students can view the lectures at any time on a computer with Internet access.

Accessories

Media centers and computer or learning labs may be available to provide faculty and students with access to additional hardware accessories, such as DVD or Blue Ray players, laptop computers and presentation projectors, video cameras and monitors, printers, and copy machines. Also, instructors will need software downloaded to their computers and simple recording equipment to record lectures for lecture capture.

Computer testing labs, usually separate from media centers, are used for student assessments that occur in a monitored testing environment. Hours of operation and the rules and regulations for use of this equipment should be shared with students during orientation. If use of the lab or computer testing center is a requirement for course activities, instructions should be included in the course syllabus.

Software and Applications

Computer programs are available for a wide variety of uses, including graphic presentations and content delivery. Software also comes in different forms, including CD-ROMs, digital videodisks (DVDs), and licensed networked programs.

Software programs can be used for either class/coursework presentations or for student self-study. Computer-assisted instruction (CAI) programs such as case presentations, simulations, tutorials, and drills may be available in the media center for student self-study. This type of software helps students with specific skills, such as critical thinking, physical assessment, or preparation for NCLEX-RN. Computer-based applications support the needs of students by allowing them to work at their own time and pace and provide for immediate feedback of their progress. Computer programs in the form of CD-ROMs can be included with the purchase of required course textbooks, but more frequently the textbook publishers provide an associated Web site where the student registers and then is able to access textbook content and integration links. Many publishing companies are providing their text-books in an entirely online format where the book can be downloaded to a computer, iPhone, iPad, or PDA. Additional computer-program software is available for individual purchase at school or local book-stores. The school may purchase licenses for computer-software pro-grams, which are then available for use by both students and faculty on the school's computer local area network (LAN). Course or learning-management systems (LMS) provide Web-based platforms in which the structure for organizing course content and information is pro-vided. Some examples of LMSs are Blackboard, WebCT, and Desire to Learn. Illuminate is educationally based Web-conferencing software that provides a real-time or synchronous classroom for students via an Internet connection.

Programs can also be accessed from distant sites through an Internet connection. Distance learning programs use the Internet and World Wide Web for course work and course conferencing. Interactive vid-eoconferencing is a type of distance-learning technology where stu-dents at different locations can synchronously view and interact in a classroom at a remote location. Students and faculty need to become comfortable with the use of basic computer software programs such as word processing as well as database and spreadsheet programs and should have the ability to access the Internet.

Clickers

Student-response systems (clickers) uses hand-held wireless devices that enable students to give a real-time response to a question in the classroom. With this type of program, the instructor uses an Internet-based performance system in conjunction with PowerPoint slides. The PowerPoint lecture can have questions built into the content being presented. For example, as the faculty member introduces new con-tent, a question is displayed on the screen, and the students are asked to individually respond to the question using the clicker. A range of question formats can be used using this technology: multiple-choice, true/false, yes/no, and rank-ordered question formats. This technol-ogy gives the instructor feedback about what the students understand, can be anonymous, and allows students to interact with the lecture. Use of the clickers increases student engagement in the classroom.

This type of technology can also be used to record attendance, for voting, for opinion polls, or for testing. If you plan to use clickers, make sure your academic institution has the software available for faculty use. Clickers are commonly used in some programs and often students are required to purchase their own clickers for use during their courses.

Virtual Reality

The creation of virtual worlds in nursing education is increasing exponentially. Virtual worlds are particularly useful for providing experiential experiences for students that mirror real-life clinical situations. Faculty can create and set up these experiences or simulations within a virtual 3D world available on the Internet known as Second Life (http://secondlife.com). This virtual world has many applications. In a simulated hospital unit or skills laboratory, students could practice their communication skills or their skills at recording vital signs. With clinical simulations in Second Life, the faculty can provide experiences for the students that might not be easily available in a real clinical setting, such as communicating with patients about end-of-life decisions. With Second Life the faculty can give real-time lectures with feedback sessions, have interactive sessions, use group-work teaching strategies as well as individual assignments. Faculty and students interact with each other through avatars, which are graphical representation of themselves, in cyberspace. Another application is teaching using case studies involving avatars. These case studies can include patient stories, videos, and images. Grading criteria for assignments in a virtual world is no different from conventional class assignments; however, the faculty member may need to allow for the huge learning curve when students begin to use Second Life. If you are planning to use Second Life, faculty and students will need assistance from the technology support staff at their academic institution. Also, faculty members will need help to build the virtual experiences and assistance with the hardware needs such as specifications related to the servers where the virtual worlds are stored and high-speed computers. Second Life can be downloaded free from the Internet (http://secondlife.com). However, there are costs involved with designing and creating virtual worlds and maintaining Second Life.

Simulation

Learning labs in nursing schools have been expanding from low-fidelity or static simulation to high-fidelity simulators in recent years. High-fidelity human simulators (HFHS) are highly interactive computerized mannequins that are used to teach critical thinking and psychomotor skills. A HFHS is an anatomically correct mannequin that can mimic real-life patient processes such as pulses, speaking, heart and lung sounds, and breathing. In some states, simulations with the HFHS can be substituted for clinical time. Faculty must have the necessary skills and technological support in order to provide high-quality simulation experiences for student teaching and learning.

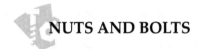

NUTS AND BOLTS

Selecting Computer Applications

Process

Using the computer is one method for delivery of course content and evaluation of student learning. Planning is essential for successful implementation of computer use in the learning process. Consulting the instruction services or similar department of the university is imperative during the planning and implementation process. This department provides support and all of the software and hardware required.

To begin the process of implementing technology, start by setting the criteria to evaluate options. The methodology and material should be presented in harmony with the rest of the curriculum. Review the program and course objectives to see if there is a good fit. Include the computer-based activities in the course objectives. Try out one new computer methodology per class or course and ask for student feedback and evaluation. Computer use requires a significant amount of time expenditure and should relate to the course credit. It also should be calculated into both student and faculty workload.

Software Content Evaluation

When assessing software for student self-study, prepare a list of content topics in the course. Be sure the content is covered with emphasis on the aspects considered most important. Also, make sure the software used in the course or for self-study is appropriate for the students. The method and content should be aimed at the level of the students in the class. Also, the school computer or media center should evaluate computer programs or software for personal use or for purchase.

Table 12.1 includes a form that could be used to evaluate computer-assisted instruction (CAI) software. This form is based on the form used earlier for evaluating a potential textbook (see Tables 8.1 and 8.2). As with the textbook evaluation, rate the elements with a Likert scale from 0 (*unsatisfactory*) to 5 (*excellent*). Other items might be evaluated simply on the basis of Yes or No.

Costs

The use of technology in instruction requires a financial investment for the institution and a significant time investment for the faculty. Adequate resources must be available to successfully use technology in course presentations. The cost will involve the need for technology support personnel, software, and hardware resources. Investments in resources must ongoing to remain technologically current.

Designing Presentations

Numerous programs are available for creating instructional programs and evaluation tools for use with students. One of the most widely used programs for developing classroom presentations is Microsoft PowerPoint. This program can be easily learned and adapted for use in various teaching situations such as classroom and Web-based presentations. As discussed earlier, PowerPoint presentations can be incorporated into student response system technology. HFHS can also be videotaped and used as part of course lecture time to teach clinical skills.

FINAL WORDS

In this age of information it is important to explore available institutional resources and to use them to enhance education. An instructional technology department should be consulted if available. In order to help students to be current and competitive as professionals, instructors should provide opportunities for them to work with computers and show them how to incorporate computers and related technology into their professional lives.

TABLE 12.1   Software Evaluation Form

Name of software_____   Author_____

Publisher_____   Publication date_____

Cost_____   Projected use_____

General:

_____   Compatible conceptual framework

_____   Comprehensive coverage of content

_____   Emphasis on nursing models

_____   Approach to nursing process consistent with course objectives

_____   Definitions consistent with course content

_____   Builds on prerequisite content

_____   Aimed at students in upper division

_____   Nonsexist and nonstereotyped language

_____   Easy to access and download software if needed

_____   Amount of equipment needed

_____   Compatible with other software used

_____   Requires utilizing instructional services

Usability:

_____   User friendly

_____   Low cost

_____   Flexible

_____   Time commitment not prohibitive

_____   Facilitates student interaction

_____   Clear instructions for getting started and working through the CAI

_____   Student can progress at own pace and skip sections if desired

_____   Immediate feedback to student

_____   Clear instructions for exiting program; student may exit whenever
         desired

_____   Built-in self-assessments or quizzes for students

_____   Web site intuitive and easily assessable

Support materials:

_____   Available Web-based instructors' manuals

_____   Available Web-based student manual

_____   Instructions only, not for purchase

_____   For individual purchase

         Cost _____

_____   Program-driven media

_____   PowerPoint slides with audio

_____   Digital videodisk

_____   Test-item bank available

_____   Book form

_____   Computer software

Comments:

FURTHER READING

Adams, A. M. (2004). Pedagogical underpinnings of computer-based learning. *Journal of Advanced Nursing, 46*(1), 5–12.

Arundell, F., & Cioffi, J. (2005). Using a simulation strategy: An educator's experience. *Nurse Education in Practice, 5*(5), 296–301. doi:10.1016/j.nepr.2005.03.001

Blake, H. (2010). Computer-based learning objects in healthcare: The student experience. *International Journal of Nursing Education Scholarship, 7*(1), Art. 16. doi:10.2202/1548–92X.1939

Brown, D., & Chronister, C. (2009). The effect of simulation learning on critical thinking and self-confidence when incorporated into an electrocardiogram nursing course. *Clinical Simulation in Nursing, 5*, E45–E52. doi:10.1016/j.ecns.2008.11.001

Chandra, V., & Chalmers, C. (2010). Blogs, wikis and podcasts: Collaborative knowledge building tools in a design and technology course. *Journal of Learning Design, 3*(2). Retrieved from http://www.jld.qut.edu.au/publications/vol3no2/documents/ChandraJLDvol3no2_000.pdf

Conlon, M., & Pavlika, V. (2009). A discussion of video capturing to assist in distance learning. *Lecture Notes in Computer Science, 5621*, 432–441. doi:10.1007/978–3-642–02774–1_47

Jeffries, P. (2007). *Simulation in nursing education.* New York: National League for Nursing.

Knobel, M., & Lankshear, C. (2009). Wikis, digital literacies, and professional growth. *Journal of Adolescent & Adult Literacy, 52*(7), 631–634. doi:10.1598/JAAL.52.7.8

Long, S. R., & Edwards, P. B. (2010). Podcasting: Making waves in millennial education. *Journal for Nurses in Staff Development, 26*(3), 96–101. doi:10:1097/NND.ObO13e318199a6f

McConnell, E. A. (2000). High-tech learning means more access, more participation, and more nurses. *Nursing Management, 11*, 49.

McRae, M. E., & Elgie-Watson, J. (2010). Using audience response technology in hospital education programs. *Journal of Continuing Education in Nursing, 41*(7), 323–328. doi:10.3928/00220124

Pinder-Grover, T., Mllunchick, J. M., Bierwert, C., & Shuller, L. (2009, June). Leveraging screencasts to strategically clarify unclear material science concepts. *Proceedings of the ASEE Annual Conference and Exposition, Austin, TX* . Code 77079.

Wiecha, J., Heyden, R., Sternthal, E., & Merialdi, M. (2010). Learning in a virtual world: Experience with using Second Life for medical education. *Journal of Medical Internet Research, 12*(1). doi:10.2196/jmir.1337

13

Guiding Independent Study

U ndergraduates in their junior or senior years and graduate
students are often ready to study a topic that is not part of the
regular curriculum. Students desire other formats of learning outside the traditional classroom setting as a result of other life
goals and responsibilities. The names given to these activities vary
from one university or college to another and often are called *directed
readings, special studies,* or *special topics.* Regardless of what they are
called, the two basic types of independent study are directed readings and a special activity of some sort. Those are the two types of
independent study that will be discussed in this chapter. It is beyond
the scope of this book to deal with such a major independent study
as a thesis.

Just how independent is independent study? Both the student and
faculty member have responsibilities when engaged in independent
study. Successful independent study experiences are dependent on the
learner's readiness to learn and their ability to learn independently. The
independent nature of self-directed learning requires critical thinking
skills, as students are in charge of their own learning throughout the
independent-study activity. The student's readiness to learn independently, as well as their learning style, must be considered when discussing the student's goals for accomplishing the independent-study
activity. The student is responsible for determining the topic to be
addressed and objectives to be accomplished. The faculty member
changes from provider of learning to the facilitator of learning and is
therefore responsible for helping to provide structure and guidance as

well as a format in which the student will accomplish the learning goals and receive credit.

GOALS

The principal goal of independent study is to promote autonomy of the student. Independent study helps to provide unique learning experiences that may not be included in the regular curriculum. It provides students with opportunities to engage in in-depth exploration of their chosen specific topic.

TOOLS

Directed Reading

Directed reading involves a student and a faculty member working out a program of reading. Generally, the student identifies a particular area of interest that usually relates to the faculty member's field of expertise. The faculty member guides the student on where to look for appropriate readings in order to meet the student's objectives. The faculty member may have to spend time teaching the student the necessary skills for searching the literature and also review with the student the ways to critique the literature and to organize the critique findings. Plan to meet with the student weekly to provide the student with feedback on his or her progress with the assignment and to ensure that expectations are being met. Regular meetings, particularly at the beginning of the directed reading, will help to keep the student on track and reduce anxiety. Also, the faculty member can assess the student's workload based on the quantity of literature retrieved (see Table 13.1).

Special Study

Special studies include all those activities outside of directed reading. This would include observational experiences, clinical practice, small research studies, and development of innovative virtual activities, among other activities. These activities require faculty to explore unique learning experiences with the student that encourage reflection and analysis of the planned experience (see Table 13.2).

TABLE 13.1   Plan for Directed Reading

Objective: To identity the nursing indications for the use of the specific concentration of epinephrine for the correct patient condition

Outcomes:

1. Identify the dose of the specific concentration of epinephrine (1:1,000 or 1:10,000 1mg/0.1mg/mL), indications for use of each concentration, and recommendations for close monitoring and management of the patient.
2. Identify appropriate nursing interventions to be implemented prior to and after drug administration.
3. Make a guide incorporating indications, effects, and related interventions.

Activities:

1. Read two to three articles per week.
2. Summarize each article.
3. Meet with faculty member for 2 hours every other week.

Evaluation:

Two hours of credit will be awarded for successfully achieving the outcomes listed above.

Agreed to by:

Student signature_____   Faculty signature_____   Date: _____

NUTS AND BOLTS

Getting Started

Meet with the student to discuss what the student wishes to accomplish. Some students come with very specific ideas about what they want to accomplish, whereas others have only a vague notion of what they want. The ability to learn at one's own pace can make independent study an attractive option for the student. While the assumption might be that better students have more specific ideas, this is not necessarily always the case. The student's learning style and readiness for learning in this format versus the traditional lecture format will determine the student's success in accomplishing outlined goals. Encourage students to select engaging learning opportunities on which they can build and perhaps explore further in another independent study activity.

TABLE 13.2   Plan for Special Study

Objectives:

1. To practice facilitating a small group of students learning about group process concepts
2. To give feedback to promote learning in a small-group experience
3. To modify a structured group experience to meet the needs of the group

Outcomes:

1. Student will be able to describe general principles of promoting healthy group functioning.
2. Student will be able to give constructive feedback to group members.
3. Student will be able to modify group exercises in a way that retains the purpose of the exercises and individualizes the approach to meeting the group's needs.

Activities:

1. Observe a faculty member conducting at least two exercises with a group of junior students.
2. Meet with the faculty member to discuss the process of the group.
3. Conduct four exercises with the group of junior students.
4. Meet with the faculty member prior to each exercise to discuss correct use.
5. Meet with the faculty member after each exercise to discuss group process and progress in meeting outcomes.
6. Read five assignments given by the faculty member.

Evaluation:

1. Student will meet the outcomes and describe orally to the faculty member how each has been accomplished.
2. Two hours of credit will be awarded for successfully achieving the outcomes listed above.

Agreed to by:

Student signature_____   Faculty signature_____   Date: _____

The Student With Specific Ideas

With the changing face of health care, there are many areas that may interest the student. As students progress through their program of study, the interest can vary from a specific disease process, clinical procedure, or drug to an interest in developing innovative patient teaching materials or to leadership- and career-related topics. When students begin looking into the topic of interest they may discover there a lack of information available in their immediate resources and become interested in seeking more information. Formation of specific goals and objectives with assistance from faculty will focus this type of inquiry. Activities the student might consider are papers, presentations, facilitation of groups, or clinical preceptorships. After clear goals and objectives are negotiated, a study plan is developed. This plan will include the objectives and details of the activity, with specific information on how the independent study fits the student's overall program. Also included is information on the time commitment of the faculty member and student, the meetings with the faculty member, the planned outcome of the independent study, and the grading rubric. In some institutions the faculty member must submit the study plan for approval to the student's program director. Once the plan is in place, a contract between the student and faculty is established. Table 13.1 demonstrates a student/faculty contract for this type of activity.

The Student Without Specific Ideas

Students have many different reasons for choosing independent study. Some may simply need additional credits for graduation or need to be a full-time student. Others may have additional commitments that make it difficult to enter the classroom setting. Often at the first meeting they may have only a vague idea of what they need to accomplish. Discussing areas of interest and future plans can help the student focus and aid in the decision of whether directed reading or an alternative will best help meet his or her needs.

It is important to spend time with the student narrowing the area for independent study. The activity planned should be structured so that learning is accomplished. Once a plan is made, a formal written contract between the student and faculty will provide a structure for the student. The contract clarifies the ultimate purpose of the activity and the requirements for completion of the independent study. Table 13.2 shows an example of this type of faculty/student contract.

Determination of Credit

In most settings, there is a range of possible credits that may be offered for the categories of independent study. That range usually is 1 to 4 credits. Some students request a certain amount of credit, and that should be considered when formulating the plan. Other students do not have a particular amount of credit in mind. During negotiations about the assignment, the student determines the amount of work he or she is willing to put into it, and that will determine the amount of credit.

The school or university may have some stipulations about the amount of time the student and the faculty member must put into the independent-study activity. Check for any policies concerning that. Such policies should be kept in mind when calculating the amount of work involved in other determinations for credit. It is typical that lecture credit is on the basis of 1 hour of lecture per week for each credit (in a semester system). Clinical and laboratory experiences are usually 3 hours a week for each credit. In addition, there are 2 to 3 hours of preparation or writing outside of class for each credit per week.

Using this information, it would be appropriate to expect the student to devote at least 3 hours a week per credit to the independent study. Part of the initial planning with the student should include making this point so the student has an adequate idea of the commitment expected. In the case of a directed reading a consideration might be how long it will take to research the topic adequately when assigning the number of credits. If the student has a certain number of credit hours to fulfill, then the amount of work to achieve that goal should be determined and made clear to the student.

Setting Objectives

The next step is for both the student and the faculty member to set objectives. Some situations may call for several objectives, whereas others may be met with a few or only one objective.

Approach

After setting objectives, a decision is made as to how the student can best achieve their learning objectives. In the case of directed reading, a plan could be made to research and extrapolate the necessary information as well as to discuss the evaluation of the objectives. In the case of an activity, an agency, a case manager or another faculty member may participate in the student's planned activity.

If a student requests an observational or clinical experience, it may take more time to identify where the student could accomplish this.

Negotiations with individuals or agencies to permit the student to observe certain activities will be necessary. It is best to work with the agencies or facilities with an observational contractual relationship with the college or university, as this will ease the negotiation process and time involved making the arrangements. Working with an agency or facility that has no relationship with the academic institution is very time-consuming, and the semester may be almost over before you receive permission for the student to have their independent experience in that setting. It may be a good use of the faculty member's time to check if there is another agency with a contractual agreement that may be willing to provide the type of experience the student has requested. A description specifying the student's role in the situation and the goals to be accomplished must be written (e.g., "For this experience, the role of the student is simply to observe and not to give patient care"). Additionally, contact information of the faculty member who is guiding the student's experience must be given to the agency. Likewise, the faculty member must receive the name of the agency employee supervising the experience.

If a student requests a specific clinical experience, determine and work out an appropriate setting for this to take place and provide or arrange for adequate supervision. In the past, providing this sort of independent study in the past was complicated, as the time involved was sometimes too prohibitive to make it possible. This has since changed, and many facilities are welcoming students into these settings, not only as a learning opportunity for the student, but also for possible recruitment purposes. An example of this type of activity might be a student interested in the emergency room or another critical-care setting where close supervision is necessary. The student may be assigned to work with a charge nurse or staff nurse who agrees to act as a preceptor. The student provides care to patients under the supervision of the nurse with the agency's approval. To further enhance the student's experience, any opportunity to observe the role of a senior leader beyond the charge nurse's role may prove beneficial to the learning experience. The student would keep a journal, reflecting on the experiences during clinical time and discuss those with the preceptor. At the end of the student's experience, a final paper or presentation detailing the experience is submitted to faculty.

Supervision

The amount of supervision required is determined by the nature of the independent study. Directed reading requires no direct supervision, but it is typical to meet with the student on a regular basis to discuss the readings. With an undergraduate, there is an expectation that summaries of the articles with some higher level processes will be prepared, such as synthesis or evaluation of the articles. With graduate students, the use of high-level processes should be expected more than simply presenting summaries.

Supervising a special study is more complex and requires more faculty time than supervising directed reading. If the experience is observational, meet regularly with the student to discuss his or her observations and to relate them to the objectives for the experience. With a clinical experience, a faculty member may directly supervise the student. If the student is assigned to be with a preceptor, meet regularly with the student and plan periodic contacts with the preceptor. Regular visits to the clinical site are recommended to see the student in the learning environment. These visits provide opportunities for the student, preceptor, and faculty member to interact and reflect on the independent-study experience.

Evaluation

As with all learning experiences, the evaluation is based on the student's ability to meet the objectives that were set. Usually, independent-study credit is based on a pass/fail. Even so, the faculty member and the student need to agree on the work that must be completed in order to receive credit. Procrastination may occur and can lead to a lack of performance in independent study. This should be handled in the same manner as if it were a traditional course. If the student is not doing the work early in the semester, advise the student to drop the course. If the work is insufficient at midterm to indicate to you that the student will be able to complete the work required, give the student a deficiency notice. A new agreement with the student regarding a time frame when the work will be completed will then be needed in order for the student to proceed with the learning activity.

In evaluating the actual performance by the student, use the criteria for similar work in other courses. For example, if the student is writing a paper, apply the criteria used in other courses the student might take at the same point in the curriculum. If the student is performing in a clinical setting, expect the same level of performance as in clinical courses at the student's level.

Evaluating students who have participated in predominately observational experiences will depend on the level of objectives that were set. For example, if the student was observing in order to synthesize information, the student would need to demonstrate orally or in writing that this has occurred. An evaluation by the preceptor assigned to the student in the clinical setting is also required.

WORDS TO THE WISE

In some academic settings, part of the determination of workload may include credit for the time spent in independent study, be sure to negotiate for the hours involved when your contract is considered. If there is an expectation to supervise students in independent study without this being figured into your contracted number of hours, negotiate with your dean or director for release time from other responsibilities such as committee work or some teaching responsibilities. Supervising independent study is not as demanding as some aspects of teaching, but if done right it takes a lot of time. Be sure to take care of yourself and get credit for it in some way, either in money or time. The rewards for such an undertaking may be the privilege of observing a student discovering a different career path as a result of the independent-study activity.

FINAL WORDS

Many individuals returning to college have full-time commitments to family and careers, and self-directed learning provides the opportunity to accomplish life, career, and educational goals.

Independent study gives students a chance to design learning experiences for themselves at the pace where they are comfortable and confident. Supervising students in directed readings or other special studies gives faculty a change of pace, in addition to assisting students to accomplish their goals in a manageable format.

FURTHER READING

Belcher, J. V., & Vonderhaar, K. L. (2005). Web-delivered research-based nursing education for seeking magnet status. *Journal of Nursing Administration, 35*(9), 382–386.

A NUTS-AND-BOLTS APPROACH TO TEACHING NURSING

Bradley, C., Erice, M., Halfer, D., Jordan, K., Lebaugh, D., Opperman, C., et al. (2007). The impact of blended learning approach on instructor and learner satisfaction with preceptor education. *Journal for Nurses in Staff Development, 23*(4), 164–170.

Buckley, S., Coleman, J., Davison, I., Khan, K. S., Zamora, J., Malick, S., et al. (2009). The educational effects of portfolios on undergraduate student learning: A best evidence medical education (BEME) systematic review. BEME Guide No.11. *Medical Teacher, 31*(4), 282–298. doi:10.1080/01421590902889897

Cleary, M., & Freeman, A. (2005). Self-directed learning and portfolio development for nurses. *Contemporary Nursing, 20,* 14–20.

Jerlock, M., Falk, K., & Severinsson, E. (2003). Academic nursing education guidelines: Tool for bridging the gap between theory, research and practice. *Nursing and Health Sciences, 5,* 219–228.

Kanwar, M., Irvin, C. B., Frank, J. J., Weber, K., & Rosman, H. (2010). Confusion about epinephrine dosing leading to iatrogenic overdose: A life-threatening problem with a potential solution. *Annals of Emergency Medicine, 51*(4), 341–344.

Levett-Jones, T. L. (2005). Self-directed learning: Implications and limitations for undergraduate nursing education. *Nurse Education Today, 25,* 363–368.

Myrick, F., & Yonge, O. (2004). Enhancing critical thinking in the preceptorship experience in nursing education. *Journal of Advanced Nursing, 45*(4), 371–380.

O'Shea, E. (2003). Self-directed learning in nurse education: A review of the literature. *Journal of Advanced Nursing, 43*(1), 62–70.

Pierson, M. A., & Schuelke, S. A. (2009). Strengthening the use of evidence-based practice: Development of an independent study packet. *The Journal of Continuing Education in Nursing, 40*(4), 171–176.

Profetto-McGrath, J. (2003). The relationship of critical thinking skills and critical thinking dispositions of baccalaureate nursing students. *Journal of Advanced Nursing,* 43(6), 569–577.

Slider, N. J., Noell, G. H., & Williams, K. L. (2006). Providing practicing teachers classroom management professional development in a brief self-study format. *Journal of Behavioral Education, 15,* 215–228.

Zadvinskis, I. M. (2008). Increasing knowledge level of evidence-based nursing through self-directed learning. *Journal for Nurses in Staff Development, 24*(4), E13–E19.

14

Helping Students to Improve Their Writing Skills

Although it is common for nursing faculty to assign papers to meet course requirements, students often are unable to meet the expectations of such assignments. The details about how to design the requirements for a paper as a major assignment are given in Chapter 9. This chapter deals with how to help students develop writing skills to make them better writers.

College students generally take one or two courses in English composition. Although they should learn the basic skills related to grammar and composition in these courses, students need continued practice to develop the ability to write effectively. The ideal way to carry this through the nursing major is for the faculty to agree on what kinds of writing their graduates should be able to do and where they need to learn to write what they need to write. In addition, it is helpful to students if the school of nursing or nursing program provide common instructions for written papers and the adoption of a particular writing style, such as that shown in the *Publication Manual of the American Psychological Association*.

GOALS

The principal goal for helping students to become better writers is to improve their ability to communicate the knowledge they will acquire. Good writing is an essential skill for the registered nurse, who must be able to write clear and accurate patient notes. Nurses throughout their career will be involved in writing policies, procedures, reports, and evaluations—all areas in which good writing skills are essential.

TOOLS

Clear Assignment

To write well, the student needs to understand what the assignment is. Establish the objectives the student is supposed to meet with the writing assignment. Make clear the important points that the student should address.

Guidelines to Give the Student

Help students improve their writing by giving them some guidance and support in mastering the process of putting ideas on paper. Present these ideas in class, or offer an extracurricular time to cover these points.

Preparing to Write

Tell the students to start by outlining the content to be covered. The main topics in the outline will suggest subheadings for the paper. Leave room in the outline to insert additional content as needed. Show them a sample outline. (Table 14.1 shows an outline of a specific topic.) Some students may be visual learners and prefer to draw a diagram linking their ideas together. This can be a rough drawing with the main idea at the center and the lesser ideas linked to it. The lesser ideas can be prioritized according to the order the student plans to put them in the paper.

Help the students to decide where to spend their preparation time in terms of how the assignment will be evaluated. In some assignments, the emphasis is on the content produced. For example, the paper may be a review of the literature on a certain topic. Other assignments focus on describing a process, such as a nursing care study. More care may be taken in presenting the content-oriented paper in scholarly tones.

TABLE 14.1   Outline for Writing a Paper

Clients Who Split: Borderline Personality Disorder

1. Introduction
   a. Childhood disruptions
      Inconsistent parenting
      Promotion of negative self-concept
   b. Characteristics
      Impulsive
      Manipulative/Internal conflicts
      Clinging/distancing
      Dependence/independence

2. Problems for nursing intervention
   a. Acting-out behavior: sexual promiscuity, substance abuse, temper tantrums, suicidal threats and gestures
   b. Manipulative behavior: splitting, blaming, helplessness
   c. Relationship behavior: yo-yoing, clinging, distancing
   d. Impulsive behavior: running away

3. Nursing interventions
   a. Firm, consistent, positive attitude
   b. Expect appropriate behavior
   c. Foster development of trust
   d. Constructive confrontation
   e. Encourage verbalization of feelings
   f. Reinforce efforts at individuation
   g. Set firm limits on manipulation
   h. Teach coping with reality problems
   i. Maintain frequent, open communication among staff to provide consistent approach

4. Description of client with examples

5. Summary

On the other hand, a process-oriented paper can be written in the first person. Faculty can improve clarity for students by using a grading rubric for the writing assignment that provides the criteria and weight of different portions of the assignment. Students can use this weighting to decide on the number of pages or paragraphs needing to be assigned to each aspect of the rubric. (See an example of a rubric in Chapter 9.)

Practicing Writing

The only way to learn to write well is by practicing. Encourage students to start by writing whatever they can think of that fits the writing assignment. Initially, they should not worry about where to start or how the material is organized. As they have ideas for a section, they should start a new page and write what they are thinking. After they have written for a while, they should leave their written work alone for a few days. When they read it again, they may see grammatical errors or problems in composition they overlooked when it was fresh. Then they should rewrite the paper, cleaning up errors and paying more attention to grammar and organization. As they read more about the topic, they will have more ideas for what they are writing. They should then set it aside again for a few days.

Although what they have written may seem rough, they are ready to ask someone else to read it. Reading drafts of the students' papers is time-consuming, but it may be possible to allocate time to read at least a page or two of each one. Reading the drafts gives faculty indications about the student's progress and provides opportunity to give students some constructive suggestions for improving their papers before they get to the final draft. Additionally, assigning peer reviewers within the class can be a helpful activity for students, with the peer review being shared with the faculty member.

Students might also ask other people to read and critique what they wrote. They should explain why they are practicing and provide the ground rules for how much feedback they really want. However, to gain as much as they can from the experience, they should give their readers as much latitude as possible to critique the work. They should ask their readers not only to say what they do not like but also ask them to provide some suggestions.

Encourage Reading

Suggest to students that they spend time reading well-written books, perhaps their favorite classic. Reading some of the classics will renew the students' acquaintance with good sentence structure and nice turns of phrases. Also, they will read material that contains correct uses of grammar. Peer-reviewed nursing journals are another good source of reading material. Students can use them to become familiar with the organization of material in a nursing context and see the importance of good writing skills in nursing. Reading their text-books, especially case studies and short essay formats, will be beneficial also.

Coping With Negative Experiences

Students can become discouraged if they are unsuccessful the first time they try to write a good paper. Often they are sensitive to criticism about their writing skills because they feel that they are not relevant to the nursing content and therefore should not be considered in part of the grade. They may be angry and feel that their writing skills have got them this far and now they are being told that they need to improve their writing, of all things! The role of the faculty member is to be supportive of the student while stressing the importance of good writing skills in nursing.

After freshman English courses, nursing students usually have no courses requiring formal writing. Then, suddenly, they are in one of their major courses, and they not only have to convey information about what they did for a patient, but they have to convey it skillfully. Because they have not been practicing this skill, nursing students may have forgotten a lot of what they have learned.

Innovative Ways to Improve Writing Skills

Faculty members may have assignments that focus on organization and presentation of ideas rather than on nursing content. This type of assignment gives students more time to concentrate on their writing skills and to pay attention to grammar and sentence structure. These assignments can be short, weekly, Web-based journal-type entries that are written and posted for the faculty member on the course management system. Timely feedback from the faculty member is important so that the students can improve their writing skills in the next journal entry. Internet-based journals will likely appeal to students who are most comfortable with the technology. Unfortunately, technology also has a downside because the insurgence in texting means that students will probably abbreviate their words and rarely write full sentences. Students may find it helpful to use some of the online programs available to practice writing or to enroll in online grammar refresher course. When helping students improve their writing skills, the faculty member must build on the students' skills and technological expertise so that the students are excited about the activities rather than seeing improvement of writing skills as an additional burden.

NUTS AND BOLTS

Guidelines for Writing Well

Use these suggestions to assist students with improving their writing skills.

Guidelines for better writing:

1. Make and follow an outline.
2. Use simple declarative sentences.
3. When in doubt about how something sounds, throw it out.
4. Avoid pretentious touches such as literary quotations that do not advance the reader's understanding of your subject.
5. Avoid slang and other colloquialisms.
6. Stop once the point is made.
7. Improve a cumbersome, ambiguous, or confusing sentence by either (a) breaking it up into more than one sentence, (b) shortening it rather than adding to it, or (c) dropping it altogether.
8. Use the same tense throughout, unless there is a particular reason to do otherwise.
9. Make sure the subject and verb of each sentence agree in number.
10. Avoid sexist language.
11. Use the third person in formal papers, unless the situation calls for a first-person account.
12. Start writing and putting ideas together without worrying about how it sounds. Polish it later after getting down the gist of the ideas and points.
13. After writing something, leave it alone for a few days. Then reread it and polish it.
14. If you are unsure of the spelling of a word, look it up in the dictionary. Spell check your finished document if using the computer.
15. The greater the sense of accomplishment upon completing the first draft of a work, the greater the need for revision.

16. If experiencing trouble writing a first sentence, start somewhere else.
17. If experiencing trouble writing a last sentence, you have probably already written it.
18. Write something every day, even if it is not directly related to your major writing project.
19. Do not be afraid to let someone read and edit the paper. Make sure the person has the expertise to critique the content and style.
20. Get one or two handbooks on English to help answer questions about syntax, grammar, and usage.
21. Make sure your paper has an introduction, main section, and conclusion.
22. Break up your piece with headings, subheadings, and so on. Use underlining and italics for emphasis.
23. If using references, write your citation of the source in the same style you intend to use for the finished product. Using a computer program to manage the references is highly recommended. This not only will make the literature, citation of references, and reference page much easier to manage, it will enable the student to build a reference library for future work.

Critiquing Writing

When evaluating your students' written work, be as constructive as possible. Use positive language and phrase feedback of problem areas as areas in need of improvement. Being sensitive to the student's vulnerability as you give feedback is crucial. Advise students that developing this important skill is vital for their future in nursing while reassuring them that mastery of this skill is attainable through practice

FINAL WORDS

Writing effectively is an essential skill for nurses. Because nursing education occurs within institutions of higher learning, part of the major is becoming a well-rounded person as well as a skillful nurse. Nursing faculty members can offer a lot to students by helping them to overcome some of their negative attitudes about expressing themselves in writing.

FURTHER READING

American Psychological Association. (2009). *Publication manual of the American Psychological Association* (6th ed.). Washington, DC: Author.

Arter, J. (2000). *Rubrics, scoring guides and performance criteria: Classroom tools for assessing and improving student learning.* (ERIC Document Reproduction Service No. ED446100.)

Clay, G. (2003). Assignment writing skills. *Nursing Standard, 17*(20), 47–52.

Daggett, L. (2008). A rubric for grading or editing student papers. *Nurse Educator, 33*(2), 55–56.

Niedringhaus, L. K. (2001). Using student writing assignments to assess critical thinking skills: A holistic approach. *Holistic Nursing Practice, 15*(3), 9–17.

Roberts, S. T., & Goss, G. (2009). Use of an online writing tutorial to improve writing skills in nursing courses. *Nurse Educator, 34*(6), 262–265. doi:10.1097/NNE.0b013e3181bc740d

Strunk, W., Jr., & White, E. B. (1999). *The elements of style* (4th ed.). New York: Longman.

Index